George Gentchos, MD
Pager #: ____________________

Thieme

Dynamic Cardiovascular MRI

Principles and Practical Examples

Dominique Didier
Osman Ratib

156 Illustrations
4 Tables

Georg Thieme Verlag
Stuttgart · New York

Dominique Didier, MD
Department of Radiology
University of Geneva
24, rue Micheli du Crest
1211 Geneve 14, Switzerland

Osman Ratib, MD, Ph.D.
Department of Radiological Sciences
UCLA, B2-165 CHS, Mail Code 172115
650 S. Charles E. Young Drive
Los Angeles, California 90095-1721, USA

Bibliographic Information published by Die Deutsche Bibliothek

Die Deutsche Bibliothek lists this publication in the Deutsche Nationalbibliografie; detailed bibliographic data is available on the internet at http://dnb.ddb.de

Published in the medico-scientific book series of Schering AG.
Where reference is made to the use of Schering products, the reader is advised to consult the latest scientific information issued by the company.

Printed in Germany

Typesetting: epline, Kirchheim unter Teck
Printing: Gulde, Tübingen
Bookbinding: Druckhaus Köthen GmbH, Köthen

ISBN 3-13-133041-4 (GTV)
ISBN 1-58890-185-8 (TNY)

2 3 4 5 6

Preface

Magnetic resonance imaging has become the most important imaging technique for the diagnosis of neurological and musculoskeletal diseases. Although the first ECG-gated magnetic resonance images of the heart were produced as early as 1983, the clinical applications of cardiovascular MRI have been quite meager over the past two decades. This hesitancy for the clinical application of cardiovascular MRI has been predicated on the perceived adequacy of existing non-invasive imaging techniques along with the technological limitations and complexities of routine clinical use of MRI of the heart. In the past two to three years, these limitations have been surmounted with the introduction of reliable fast and real-time MR imaging techniques.

The authors of the current volume have been actively contributing to the development and clinical application of cardiovascular MRI during the past two decades. This book reflects their intense and long-term experience. It effectively conveys the important concepts and features cardiovascular images of extraordinary quality.

The book is being published at a fortuitous time when there is an increasing interest in acquiring practical knowledge of cardiovascular MRI among cardiac diagnosticians; moreover, the accompanying CD-ROM permits the dynamic aspects of cardiovascular MRI to be more full appreciated.

Charles B. Higgins, M. D.
San Francisco, California

Table of Contents

1 Cardiac MR Imaging Techniques

Magnetic resonance images depict cardiovascular anatomy with high spatial and temporal resolution resulting in high morphological and functional clarity [1,2]. Cardiovascular anatomy can be imaged in virtually any oblique plane. Aside from the ability to aid in the diagnosis of cardiovascular pathology, careful examination of high-resolution MR images provides an ideal in vivo imaging tool for the evaluation of human anatomy and complex anomalies. Imaging the heart and cardiovascular structures often requires particular attention to the imaging techniques and careful positioning of the imaging planes that are best suitable for particular clinical problems.

Transverse, sagittal, and coronal images are commonly preset in the standard acquisition protocols of MR scanners. This may confer an important advantage when the system is being used infrequently for cardiac imaging and the operators are less familiar with aligning scans on the basis of the intrinsic cardiac axes (see below). These imaging planes are also highly reproducible for serial follow-up evaluations in an individual patient. A comprehensive and more accurate evaluation of the cardiac cavities and great vessels usually requires additional multi-oblique planes adjusted according to cardiac anatomic markers and is highly dependent on the orientation of the heart in the thorax [3].

1.1 Standard Views in Cardiac Imaging

Cardiology investigations often rely on more than one imaging modality for a given clinical problem. Usually, cardiac images obtained from different imaging modalities are acquired in different orientations with differences in position and in image presentation. Each imaging technique has its own standard views based on the possibilities and limitations of the method of image acquisition. Echocardiographic standard views are often used as references. However, because echocardiographic standard views were established based on the most optimal acoustic window through the chest wall they are obtained in multiple-oblique planes. Other tomographic imaging techniques such X-ray computed tomography (CT) were initially more limited in the degree of freedom that usually only allowed sectional planes parallel or orthogonal to the long axis of the body.

With rapid developments of cardiac MRI imaging techniques as well as the capability for post-processing large image sets to generate sectional images in different oblique planes it is possible to obtain images in any possible orientation. A set of basic standard imaging planes of the heart has been established by international groups of specialists and published under the joint sponsorship of the American College of Cardiology, the Society of Nuclear Medicine and the American College of Radiology [4,5].

1.1.1 Orthogonal Image Plane Orientation

Standard plane orientations (Fig. 1.1) used in cardiac MRI were often based on initial imaging techniques described earlier when the MRI scanners were not capable of acquiring tomographic images along multi-oblique orientations.

Advanced MRI imaging protocols allow images to be acquired in any oblique plane which is particularly useful for cardiac imaging where image planes must be adjusted according to the axis of the heart rather than along the axis of the body. Typical standard views include a horizontal long axis plane also often referred to as a "four-chamber view" along the long axis of the heart and running from the apex to the base across the two ventricular and atrial cavities. The other standard view is the vertical long axis view perpendicular to the previous one also referred to as a "two-chamber view". The vertical long axis view can be either aligned along the left ventricle or along the right ventricle. Another standard view that is commonly used in all cardiac imaging modalities is the short axis view obtained across the heart perpendicular to the long axis and cutting through the two ventricles (Fig. 1.2). The shorts axis views can be obtained at different levels from the base to the apex of the heart.

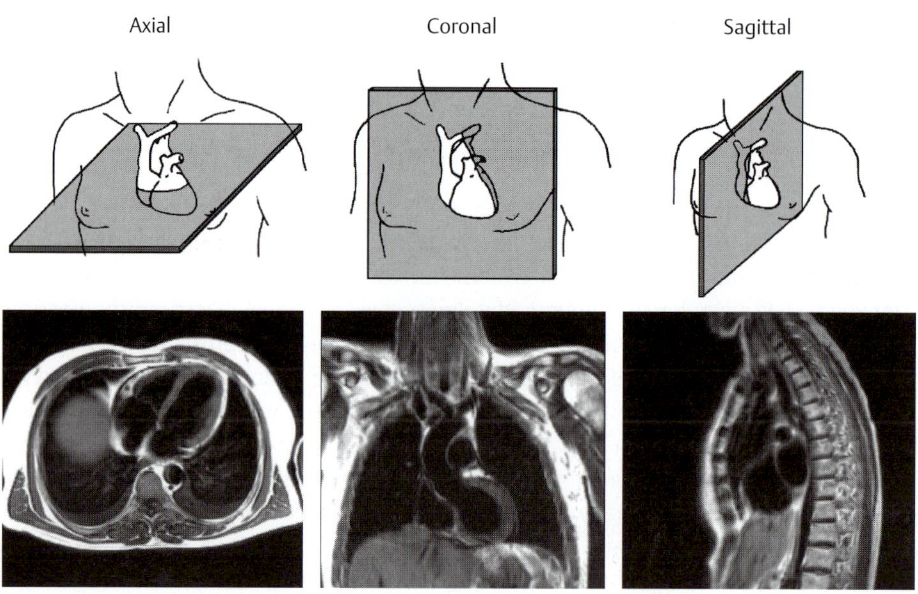

Fig 1.1 MRI standard orthogonal views: transverse, coronal and sagittal.

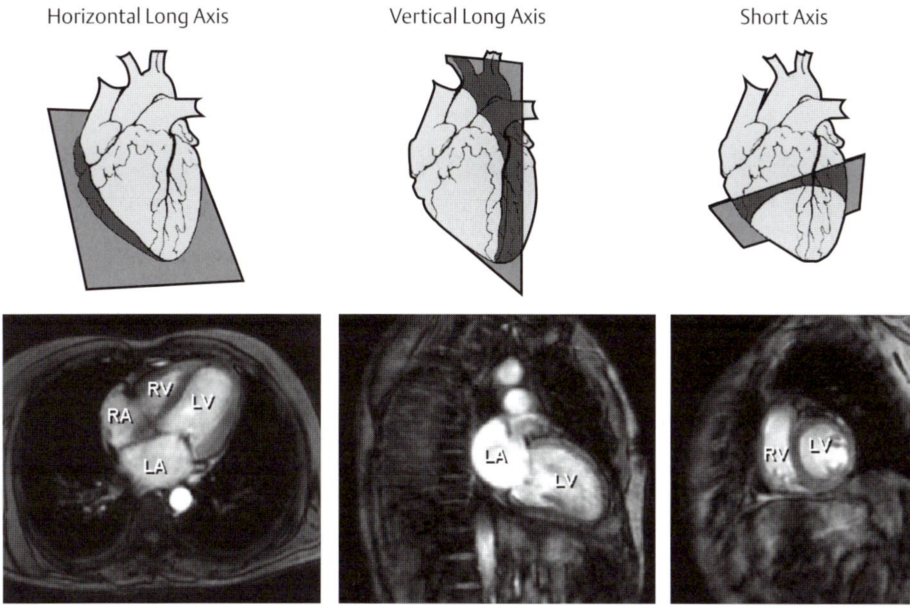

Fig. 1.2 MRI standard oblique views along the cardiac axis: vertical long axis, horizontal long axis and short axis.

1.1.2 Oblique Plane Positioning

In order to adequately acquire the standard cardiac views it is important to properly position the multi-oblique imaging planes following positioning steps that must be performed sequentially. On scanners that only allow a single view to be used as a scout image, the following steps must be executed for positioning the subsequent image acquisition (see also Fig. 1.3).

- The study should start with the acquisition of straight ***transverse*** images (also called axial slices) perpendicular to the long axis of the body.
- Using a transverse image across the heart it is possible to determine the left ventricular long axis parallel to the septum resulting in a sagittal-oblique plane. This imaging plane will be referred to as the ***vertical long axis*** plane. It corresponds to the "apical-two-cavities" view in echocardiography.
- Subsequently, a second oblique plane can be positioned on the vertical long axis view along the long axis of the LV. This resulting plane, called the ***horizontal long axis*** corresponds to the "apical-four-cavities" view in echocardiography.
- Finally the last, but probably most important, plane is the ***short axis plane***. It can be positioned either on the vertical or the horizontal long axis view (or using both long axis planes for scanners that allow multiple "scout" images). On MRI images the horizontal long axis view is preferred because it clearly shows the right ventricular cavity allowing a better positioning of the LV short axis plane at an identi-

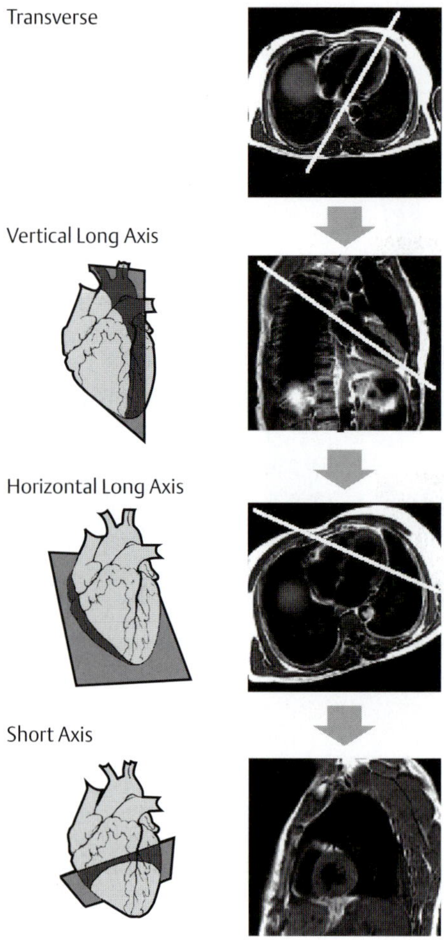

Fig. 1.**3** The sequential selection of the three standard tomographic planes that can be used in all imaging modalities. The sequence shown here is applied to MRI images.

fiable position perpendicular to the septum. The exact angular orientation of the short axis plane must be adjusted perpendicular to the septum and parallel to the atrio-ventricular valve planes.

On scanners that allow multiple scouts to be used simultaneously to position the acquisition planes it is possible to more accurately position the images along the heart axes and to account for angulations and rotations of the heart in the chest. Use of two simultaneous scout images will allow the positioning of multiple oblique images using the following steps (see Fig. 1.**4**).

- The study should start with the acquisition of straight ***transverse*** images.
- Using a transverse image across the heart it is possible to determine the left ventricular long axis parallel to the septum resulting in the ***vertical long axis*** plane.

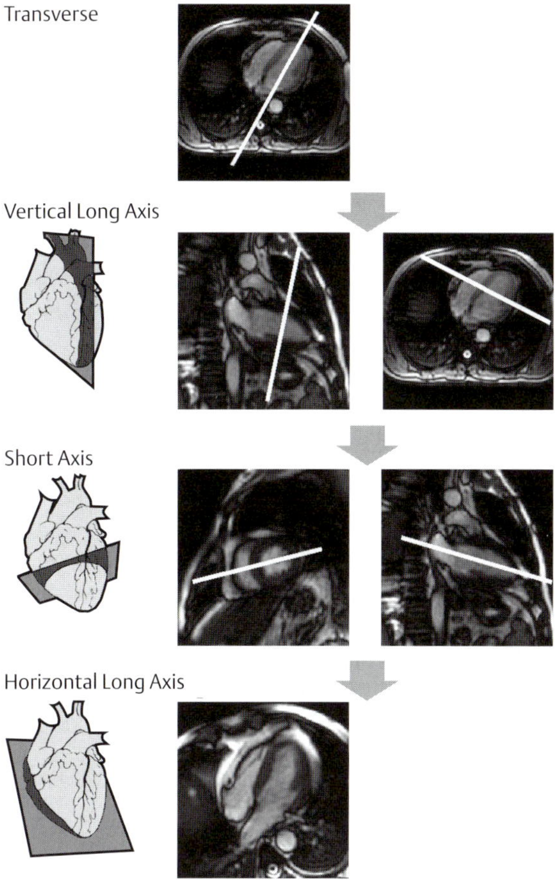

Fig. 1.4 The sequential selection of the standard multiple oblique planes using two simultaneous scout images for positioning of the imaging plane.

- Using both the axial and vertical long axis view, accurate position of ***short axis*** views can be achieved.
- Subsequently, the ***horizontal long axis*** plane can be positioned on the vertical long axis view and a short axis view.

1.1.3 Standard Orthogonal Views of the Heart

Most cardiac MRI studies will include initial sets of images acquired on one or more standard planes orthogonal to the body axis. In order to facilitate the identification of the different anatomical structures a set of annotated images obtained in the three standard orthogonal planes are shown in Figs. 1.5 to 1.7 below.

Transverse Images

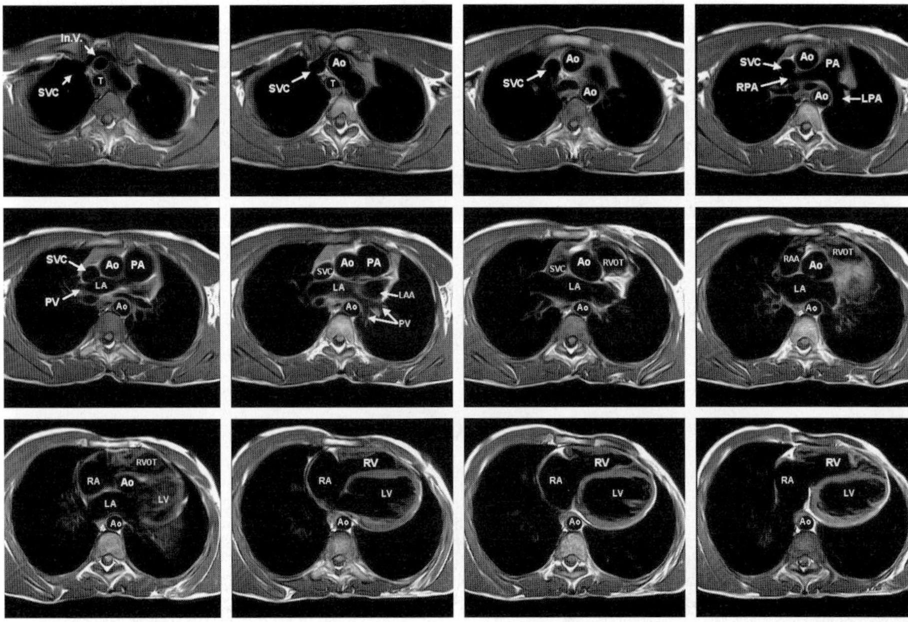

Fig. 1.**5** A set of transverse (axial) planes acquired in a normal individual.
SVC = superior vena cava, In.V = innominate vein, T = trachea, Ao = aorta, PA = pulmonary artery, RPA = right pulmonary artery, LPA = left pulmonary artery, LA = left atrium, RA = right atrium, RVOT = right ventricular outflow tract, RV = right ventricle, LV= left ventricle.

Sagittal Images

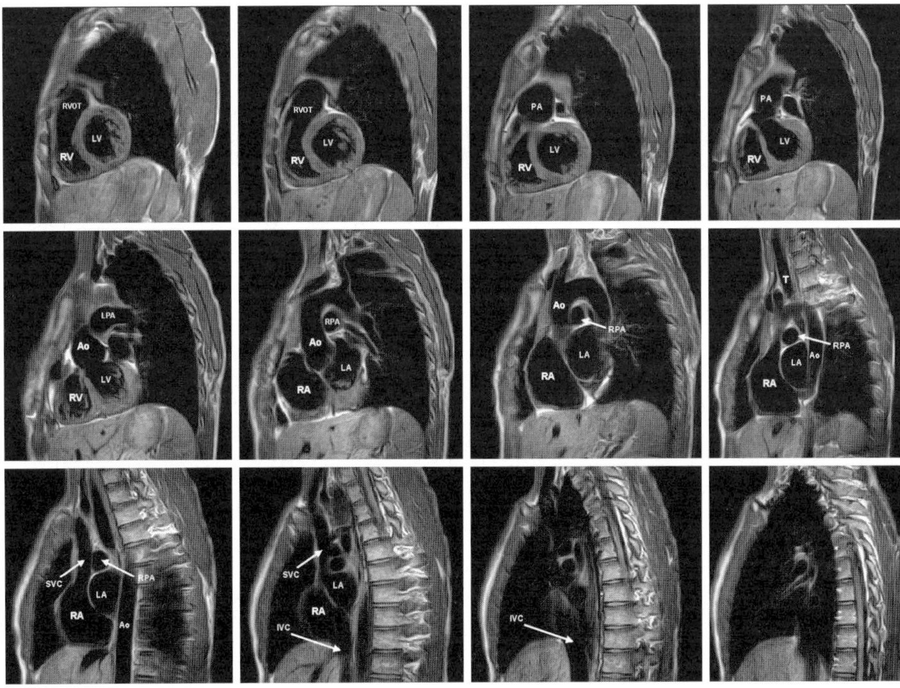

Fig. 1.**6** A set of sagittal planes acquired in a normal individual.
SVC = superior vena cava, In.V = innominate vein, T= trachea, Ao = aorta, PA = pulmonary artery, RPA = right pulmonary artery, LPA = left pulmonary artery, LA = left atrium, RA = right atrium, RVOT = right ventricular outflow tract, RV = right ventricle, LV = left ventricle, IVC = inferior vena cava.

Coronal Images

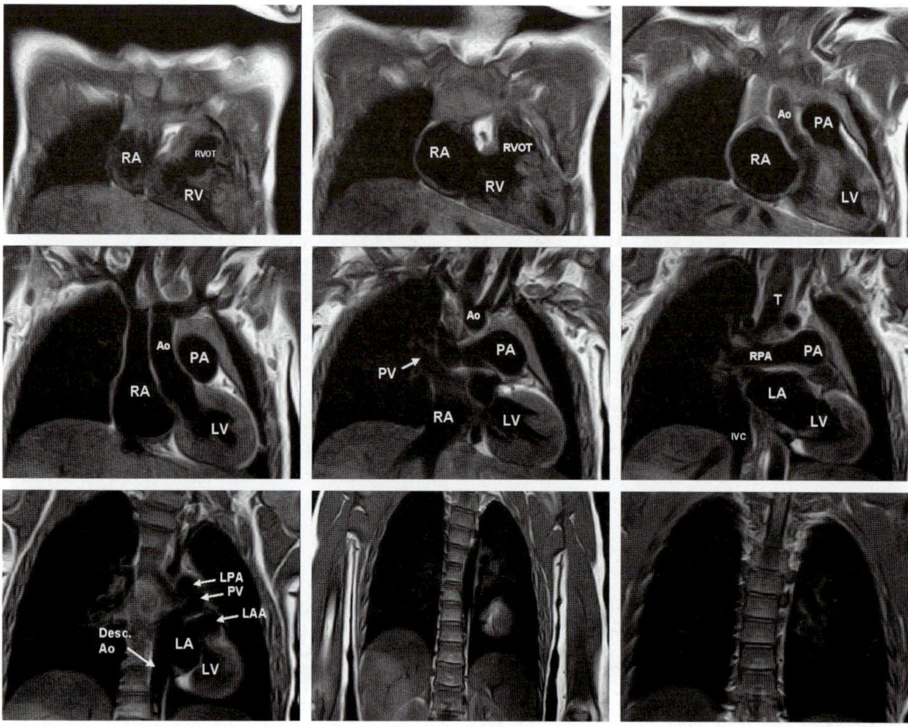

Fig. 1.**7** A set of coronal planes acquired in a normal individual.
SVC = superior vena cava, In.V = innominate vein, T = trachea, Ao = aorta, PA = pulmonary artery, RPA = right pulmonary artery, LPA = left pulmonary artery, LA = left atrium, RA = right atrium, RVOT = right ventricular outflow tract, RV = right ventricle, LV = left ventricle.

1.1.4 Oblique Cardiac Imaging Planes

Functional and anatomic evaluation of the heart and cardiac cavities requires images to be acquired in multiple oblique planes along the axes of the heart itself. This is particularly important for images acquired in dynamic (cine) mode for analysis of cardiac function, wall motion evaluation and assessment of valvular deficiencies [6,7]. The examples below illustrate the most common standard views (see Figs. 1.**2** and 1.**3** for positioning techniques of these different planes). The exact position of these planes across the heart will vary depending on the clinical requirements and the need for visualization of different anatomic structures [5]. The images in Figs. 1.**8**, 1.**9** and 1.**10** were acquired at the mid-level across the heart.

Vertical Long Axis Images (2 Chamber View)

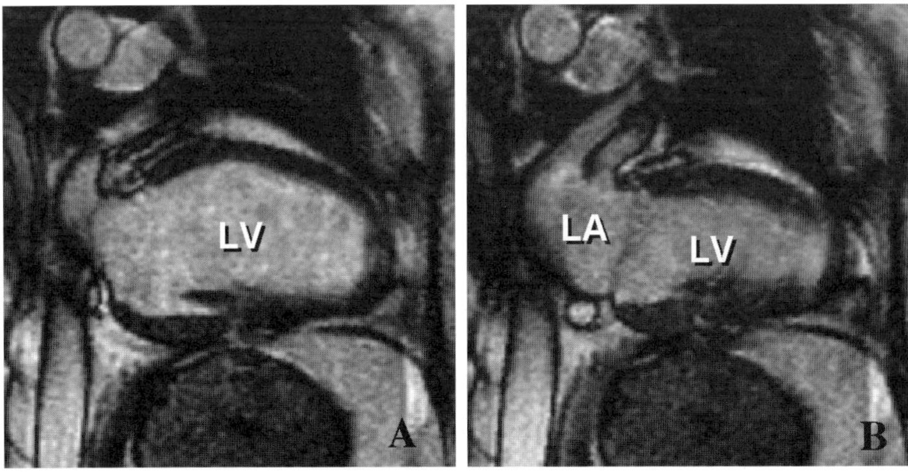

Fig 1.**8** A set of vertical long axis cine images in diastole (**A**) and systole (**B**).
RV = right ventricle, LV = left ventricle, RA = right atrium, LA= left atrium.

Horizontal Long Axis Images (4 Chamber View)

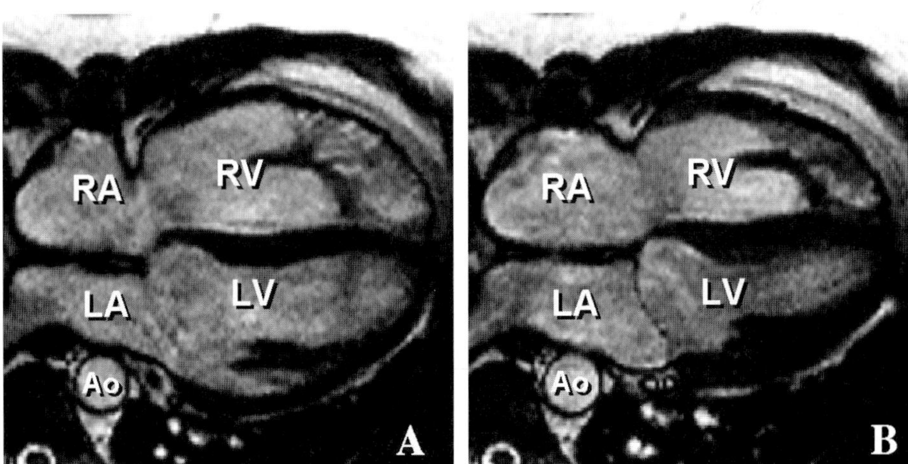

Fig 1.**9** A set of horizontal long axis cine images in diastole (**A**) and systole (**B**).
RV = right ventricle, LV = left ventricle, RA = right atrium, LA = left atrium, Ao = aorta.

Short Axis Images

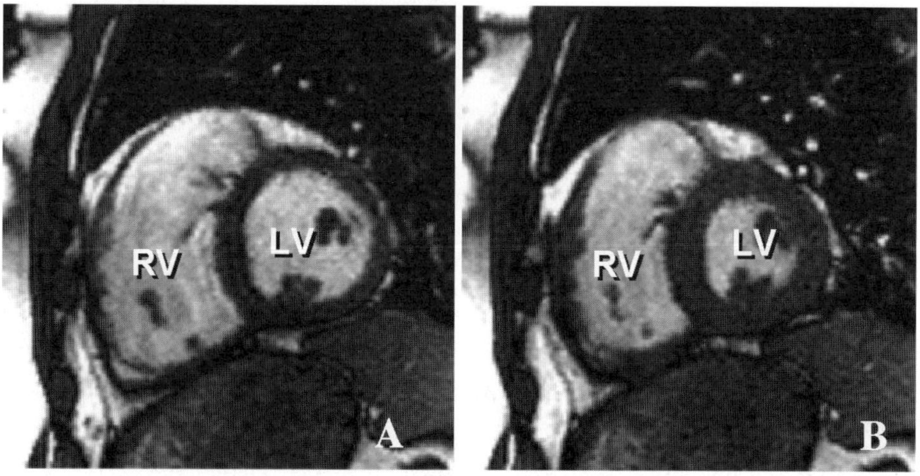

Fig. 1.**10** A set of short axis cine images in diastole (**A**) and systole (**B**). RV = right ventricle, LV = left ventricle.

An additional "long axis" view of the heart also referred to as the left ventricular outflow track (LVOT) image which is obtained from an oblique-plane positioned on a coronal image along the long axis of the heart parallel to aortic outflow track (Fig. **1.11**). This view is very similar to the parasternal long axis view of echocardiography and is particularly useful for the evaluation of aortic valve anomalies.

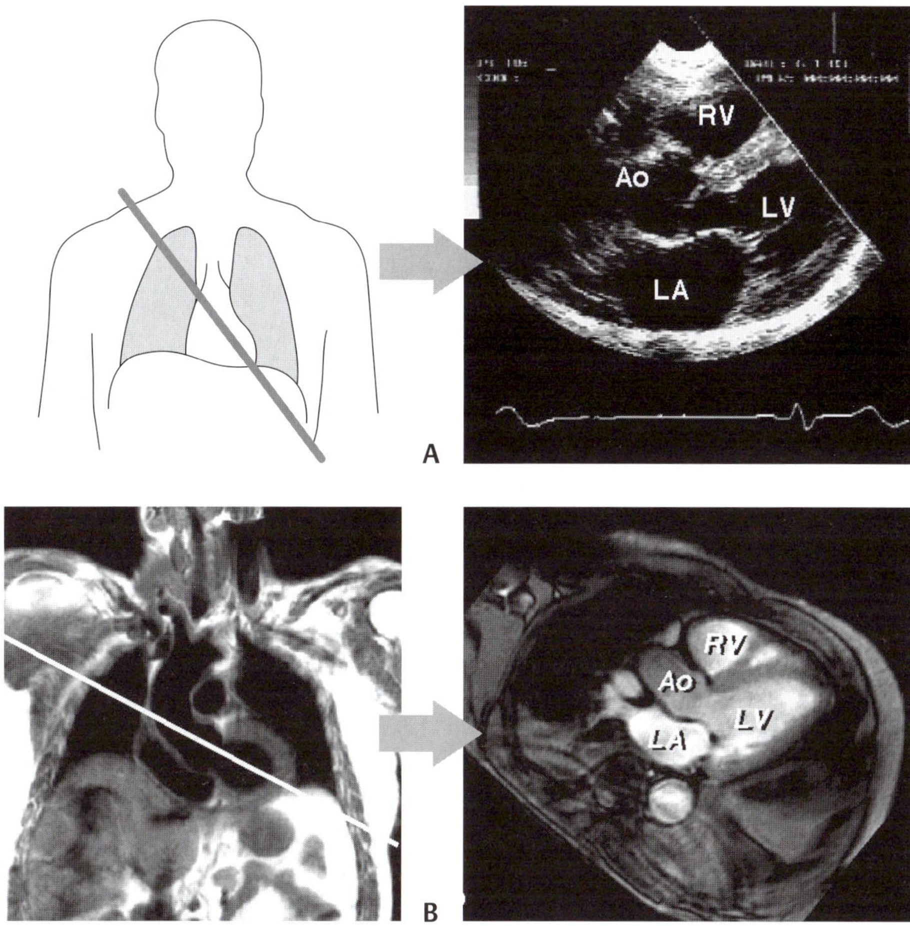

Fig. 1.**11** MRI "LVOT" plane which corresponds approximately to the parasternal long axis view of echocardiography.

1.2 Techniques and Imaging Sequences

1.2.1 Cardiac Gating (ECG Gating)

Cardiac gating uses the electrical signal detected by leads placed onto the patient's chest to trigger each imaging sequence. In this way each image is always acquired at the same phase of the cardiac cycle so that motion artifacts and blurring from cardiac motion are reduced. The quality of the ECG signal depends highly on correct placement of the leads. Accurate ECG gating is crucial to optimize image quality [8,9].

1.2.2 Lead Placement

There are usually four leads that are color-coded for easy use. Some systems may only use three leads. In addition, not all systems use the same color coding but the principle of their placement is the same. Leads can be placed either on the chest or on the patient's back. Anterior placement is usually simpler as the landmarks are easier to find. In addition, if the leads are placed posteriorly the patient lies on them during the examination, which may be uncomfortable. The anterior lead placement is described here but if the trace on the ECG monitor is poor, the leads can be placed posteriorly in a mirror image to the anterior leads. This may improve the trace. The exact positioning of the leads may vary for optimal signal recording. Some systems may not have color coding, but directions on lead placement are usually given by the manufacturer. Leads can be placed in a variety of ways as long as the above criteria are met. Fig. 1.**12** shows the simplest method of lead attachment.

The black lead may be omitted if it is not available on the system. Once the leads are attached and plugged into the system, check that the ECG trace is satisfactory. Traces vary according to rate, rhythm and cardiac output. These, in turn, depend on the activity of heart that is often altered by certain disease processes. Arrhythmia and poor cardiac output (which may be why the patient is being examined) are common problems.

If the trace is satisfactory the patient is placed within the magnet core. This action frequently alters the trace and often does so to such an extent that the trace is no longer acceptable. The commonest problem is an elevation of the T wave so that the

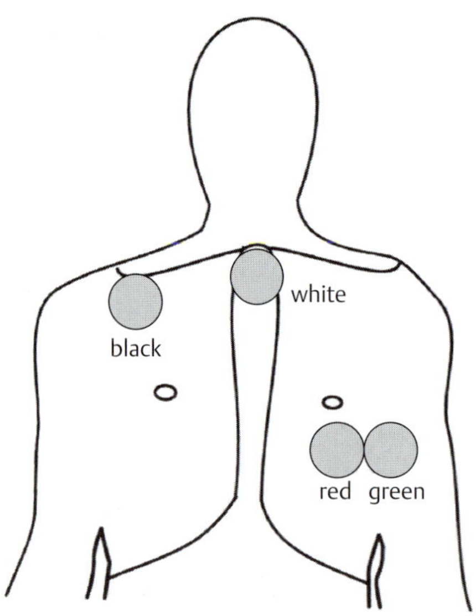

Fig. 1.**12** The correct placement of gating leads.

black lead	right upper chest below clavicle
white lead	in the midline on the superior aspect of the sternum
red lead	one intercostal space directly inferior to the left nipple
green lead	lateral to the red lead as close as possible to it but not touching it

system cannot distinguish it from the R wave. If this occurs, or if the original trace is unsatisfactory, re-positioning of the leads in different order or different locations is often required until the most optimal trace is obtained.

1.2.3 How to Improve the Trace

- Always ensure that the electrodes are firmly attached to the chest wall. In male patients shave any chest hair in the region of the electrodes and clean the skin with alcohol. This removes grease that may prevent proper attachment. After the skin is dry the electrodes are attached.
- Make sure that the leads are firmly attached to the stickers in the correct order.
- The leads may be swapped around or placed posteriorly to improve the trace. Initially swap the black and the white leads or the red and the green leads. If this fails to improve the trace, try any other variation of lead placement.

If after all these measures are taken the trace is still poor, the problem could be a faulty monitor or a software problem. Gating is often unreliable and there are occasions when the operator has to accommodate with the trace displayed or change to peripheral gating using pressure pulse detection [10] or pseudo-gating (dispensing with gating and setting a TR that is equal to the RR interval).

1.2.4 MR Imaging Sequences

It is worth reiterating that, irrespective of the imaging plane, the specific imaging sequence selected should be dictated by the clinical questions asked. A spin-echo technique is usually sufficient for defining morphology and a gradient-echo technique frequently provides complementary information. Initial, quickly acquired spin-echo images are referred to as “scouts.” They have low-to-medium resolution and are used to identify the appropriate planes for high-resolution imaging. The major trade-off for increased scan resolution is increased imaging time. As discussed above, however, increasing imaging time does not result in a linear increase in resolution. Although the signal-to-noise ratio increases, the lengthened imaging time can also result in increased artifact. Artifacts can appear to such an extent that overall image quality may not be improved.

1.2.5 Multiplanar Scout Images (Localizers)

Since the position and axes of the heart can vary significantly from one patient to another, it is always necessary to acquire a series of scout images (localizers) prior to any study. The main requirements for these scout images is that the anatomic structures are recognizable and that the acquisition time is as short as possible. Most scanners allow the acquisition of multiple scout images simultaneously in three orthogonal directions (Fig. 1.**13**). In some older systems it may be necessary to acquire

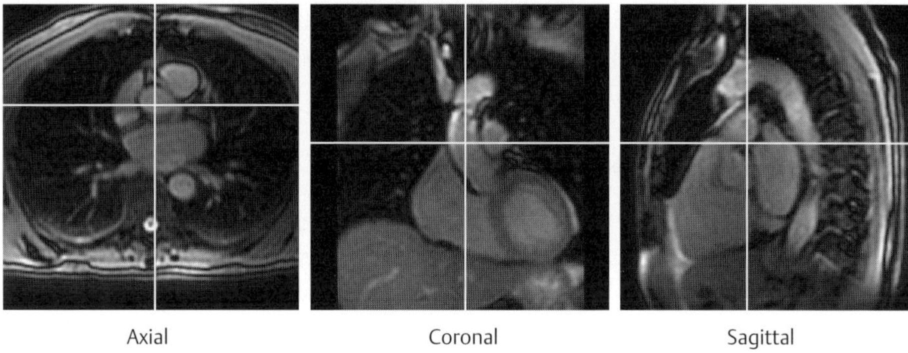

Fig. 1.**13** Typical scout images obtained in 3 orthogonal planes.

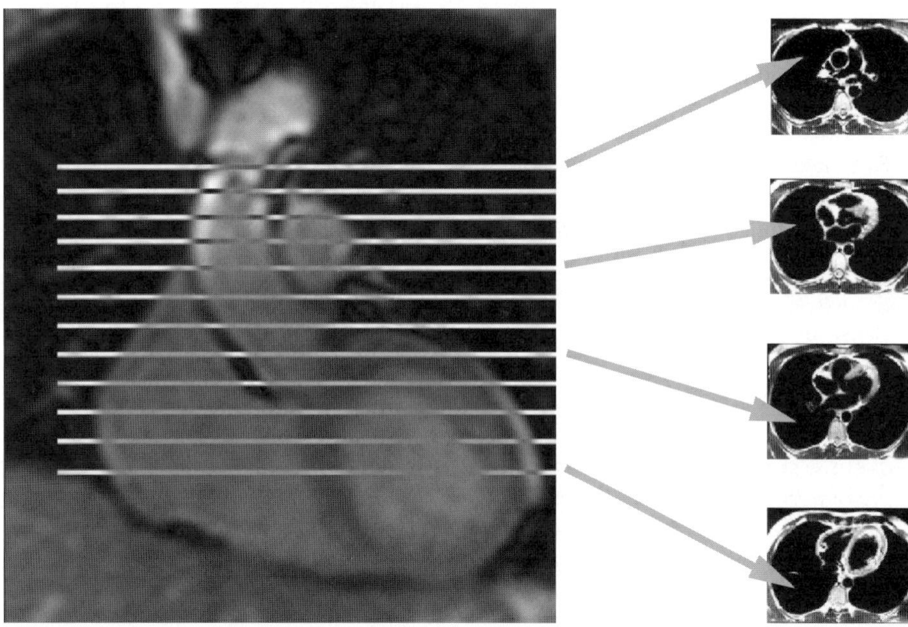

Fig. 1.**14** Positioning of axial (transverse) slices over a coronal scout image.

scout images sequentially in the three orthogonal dimensions axial, coronal and sagittal.

The scout images are then used for proper positioning of subsequent diagnostic imaging sequences (Fig. 1.**14**). They are used to adequately select the axis and range of imaging planes across the heart and anatomic structures of interest (see example below).

Subsequent images can also be positioned on images acquired sequentially. In most cases, when a multi-oblique plane is required to match the cardiac axes, it is necessary to use intermediary planes to position subsequent sequences (see example of multi-oblique positioning of images along the cardiac axes in Fig. **1.4**).

1.2.6 Cardiovascular Morphology

High spatial resolution and high image contrast are required for adequate morphological assessment of cardiac structures and thoracic vessels. All images must be acquired using ECG-gated synchronization to allow for minimal motion artifacts of the cardiac structure. Contiguous adjacent slices recorded at different phases of the heart cycle are usually acquired to minimize the acquisition time of these static images. Acquiring all images at the same phase of the heart cycle would require much longer acquisition times.

T1-weighted spin-echo (SE) sequences are most commonly used for morphological evaluation of cardiovascular anatomy. These sequences, however, may suffer from respiratory motion artifacts, even when performed with many signal averages and long TE at the cost of longer acquisition times. Fast spin-echo and turbo spin-echo (TSE) techniques reduce scan time considerably, but suffer from the same type of motion artifacts. Dark-blood-prepared TSE is commonly used with breath-hold TSE sequences.

Fast imaging sequences that are more robust with regard to motion artifacts are the half-Fourier acquired single-shot turbo spin-echo (HASTE) sequences with dark-blood preparation showing much less motion artifacts because of the short acquisition window.

1.2.7 Cardiac Function

Analysis of cardiac function and myocardial wall motion remain the key diagnostic elements of dynamic cardiac MR imaging. Gated cine sequences can be acquired in any oblique plane along the cardiac cavities or great vessels similar to echocardiographic images but with a higher spatial resolution and lesser limitation in plane positioning. Echocardiography often suffers from limitation of adequate acoustic windows for image acquisition. MRI also has a high tissue contrast allowing better delineation of myocardial and vascular structures from blood and vascular cavities. Traditionally functional evaluation of cardiac wall motion is assessed using ECG-gated gradient-echo (GE) techniques or segmented (fast) gradient-echo techniques. The resulting images are multi-phase bright-blood images depicting cardiac motion in multiple frames through the cardiac cycle. These dynamic images also provide additional information on blood flow patterns across the cardiac cavities and large vessels due to the changes in signal intensity induced by turbulent flow patterns. The changes in blood intensity with turbulent flow will depend, however, on the imaging parameters and can vary significantly with different imaging setups. Particularly with faster imaging sequences with shorter TE, the contrast of signal voids generated by

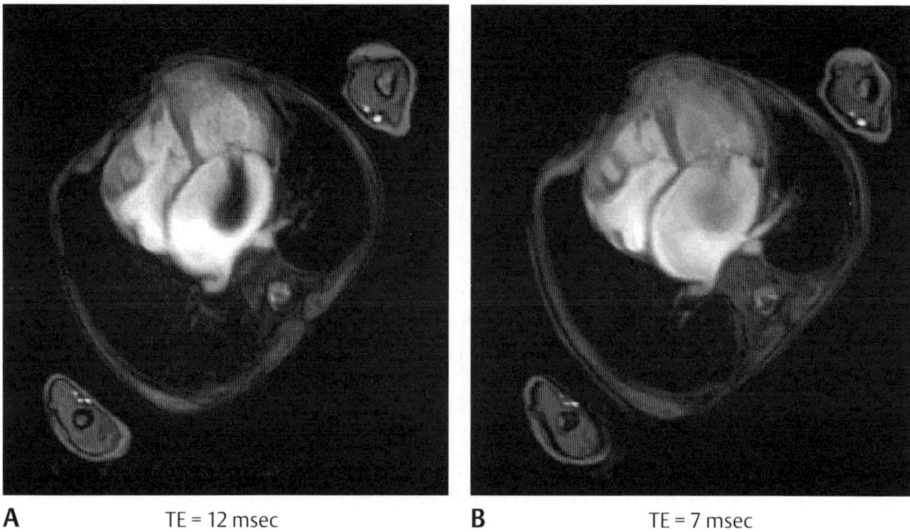

Fig. 1.**15** Example of the effect of different imaging parameters such as a shorter TE on the intensity and contrast of signal "voids" induced by turbulent flow in the case of mitral regurgitation.

turbulent flow can be significantly less prominent (Fig. 1.**15**). Shorter TE however allows for faster imaging sequences and breath-hold acquisitions.

Recent developments in new imaging sequences have led to "ultra-fast" sequences allowing high temporal resolution and very rapid acquisition of dynamic ECG-gated sequences of the heart and great vessels [11,12,13]. There are basically three different fast-imaging groups. One of these techniques utilizes multiple echoes to speed up the filling of the k-space. This technique can be applied to both SE sequences and GRE sequences. The second method consists of the preparation of the magnetization to provide higher contrast for short-TR short-TE GRE sequences. A third technique consists of acquiring only half of the k-space, the so-called half-Fourier imaging technique, which is often utilized in conjunction with the multiple-echo approach in an SE-based acquisition mode.

Segmented true-FISP (fast imaging with steady-state precession) has recently been introduced by several manufacturers as a fast, high-contrast MR imaging technique for cardiovascular applications. Recent clinical studies have demonstrated the superiority of true-FISP imaging techniques over the more commonly used segmented FLASH cine images. Fast gated, segmented FLASH sequences generally provide good quality breath-hold images with adequate temporal and spatial resolution. Spoiled gradient-echo sequences, like FLASH, rely on inflow enhancement to generate blood-to-myocardium contrast, and thus also the tendency toward blood saturation that occurs when the TR is decreased. This limits the lowest useful TR parameter that can be applied which, in turn, limits the spatial and temporal resolution. True-FISP

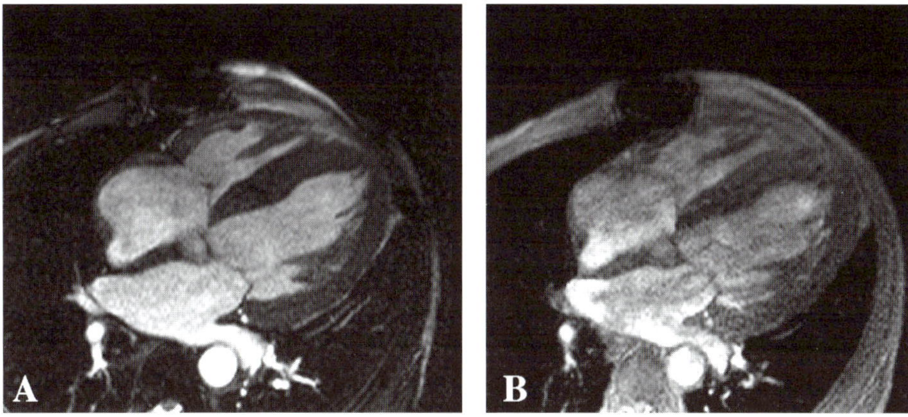

Fig. 1.**16** Comparison of dynamic cine images obtained in the horizontal long axis plane using (**A**) a gated true-FISP cine sequences and (**B**) a standard segmented gradient-echo (GE) cine sequence. Note the higher myocardium-to-blood contrast and the higher special resolution of the FISP image.

is a steady-state technique that recycles coherent transverse magnetization and the signal is determined by the T2-to-T1 signal ratio. Because blood has a significantly higher T2-to-T1 ratio than myocardium, true-FISP excellently differentiates the blood, myocardium and epicardial fat. Segmented true-FISP cine images of the heart show superior overall image quality and can be acquired in half the imaging time required for segmented FLASH images (Fig. 1.**16**). True-FISP images also better depict anatomic and functional abnormalities of the heart.

1.2.8 MR Angiography (MRA) Techniques

The early developments of MR angiography protocols were based on 2D and 3D time-of-flight (TOF) sequences [14,15]. The angiographic effect of TOF sequences is based on the principle that unsaturated blood flowing into a 3D imaging volume with primarily saturated stationary tissue will result in the blood appearing hyperintense compared to the surrounding tissues. A complementary method used to improve the contrast between the vessel lumen and surrounding tissue is the application of a magnetization transfer pulse (MTS) that increases background suppression. An alternative to 3D TOF imaging sequences is the 2D TOF sequences. The main drawback of the 3D TOF technique is the progressive saturation of blood that travels through the volume. The idea of 2D TOF is to make every slice an entry slice thus improving contrast dramatically compared to 3D TOF. The disadvantage of 2D TOF is the prolonged imaging time or the limited coverage of the sequentially applied slices. These slices have to be acquired with a significant overlap in order to compensate for the signal distortion at the edge of the slices. Otherwise a typical "staircase" pattern will appear on MIP or volume reconstructed 3D images.

1.2.9 Contrast-Enhanced MRA

With the progress in scanner development and the ability to acquire fast 3D MRA images within a breath-hold – or during the first passage of a bolus of contrast – the so-called contrast-enhanced MRA techniques have become the method of choice for visualization of the great vessels of the chest and abdomen [16–19]. Vascular visualization using Gd-enhanced 3D MRA relies on the T1 shortening of blood by contrast media during its intravascular transit. A GRE technique is applied with the shortest suitable TE, the shortest possible TR and a moderate excitation angle to provide an image of a passing bolus.

The challenging part of this technique is to adequately adapt the acquisition time to the passage of the contrast bolus in the vascular bed of interest [19,20,21]. The timing between the injection of the bolus and the start of the breath-hold acquisition is critical and should be set to acquire the central low k-space frequencies at the time the bolus passes through the region of interest. For most pulse sequences, sequential ordering of k-space is employed such that the center of the k-space is acquired during the middle or center of the imaging period. Since the central k-space determines image contrast, only vessels that are contrast-enhanced during the acquisition of central k-space will be visualized on the Gd-enhanced 3D MRA. The periphery of k-space that contributes primarily to image resolution is also important; however, its acquisition is less time-sensitive.

The exact timing of the images to coincide with the peak enhancement of the target vessels can be determined in several ways. The simplest way is using a fixed scan delay based on an "educated guess" of an average transit time across the cardiovascular circulation. For a typical 15–30 seconds acquisition sequence with a 0.2 mmol/kg contrast bolus (i.e., 30–40 ml) injected at 2 ml/sec, the imaging of the thoracic aorta should begin approximately 10 seconds after the beginning of the intravenous infusion. For pulmonary arteries, imaging should begin 2–3 seconds after contrast media injection has begun. These timing values may work fairly well on patients with normal cardiovascular transit time. They may be significantly inaccurate, however, in clinical conditions where the cardiovascular transit time is prolonged or shortened such as in severe cardiac insufficiencies or when intracardiac shunts are present.

A more accurate method for estimating the arrival time of contrast media into the target vasculature is based on the acquisition of a bolus timing scan using a 1–2 ml test bolus of contrast media [22]. This can be performed using a fast 2D gradient-echo set of images over the target structures with a rate of one image every second. These images will allow one to determine the time required for the bolus to reach the target vasculature from the site of injection. Using this information, the appropriate time delay to align the central k-space with the vascular enhanced can be calculated.

The third method for timing Gd-enhanced MRA relies on the triggering of image acquisition in real time [20, 21]. These methods, that are provided by most manufacturers on their recent scanners, allow monitoring of the signal intensity within an operator-defined region of interest encompassing part of the target vasculature to determine when to initiate data acquisition. The bolus detection using this technique has the advantage of being fully automated without the need for a test bolus injection. It also can be performed successfully with hand infusion.

To improve timing further, several investigators have proposed alternative methods of k-space phase ordering. One strategy is to acquire the central lines of the k-space early during the imaging period. This technique, called centric phase ordering, enables the acquisition of central crucial image contrast data first. This may be beneficial for imaging patients with limited breath-holding ability, ensuring that the critical central k-space data is acquired earlier during the breath-hold. Incomplete breath-holding would thus only corrupt peripheral lines of k-space and result in less significant degradation of the images. The disadvantage of this technique is due to its higher sensitivity to fluctuations in signal intensity that may occur during the arrival of the contrast media in the vessels of interest. Premature acquisition of images using a centric phase ordered acquisition may result in significant "ringing" artifacts of bright and dark bands parallel to the vessels that can render the study non-diagnostic.

For optimal image quality, thoracic MRA should be performed in a breath-hold to minimize the artifacts related to respiratory motion. Therefore, the fastest possible imaging sequence, usually a fast 3D gradient-echo pulse sequence should be used [16]. The imaging parameters and partition dimension should be carefully adjusted to achieve the smallest possible voxel size while allowing sufficient spatial coverage of the target vessels and yet still be acquired within a breath-hold. On most current scanners, a fast 3D gradient-echo sequence using the shortest possible repetition time (e.g., 4–6 msec), shortest possible echo time (e.g., 1–3 msec), and a 30–40° flip angle can be performed within 20–40 seconds. The imaging time can be decreased by using partial Fourier imaging, decreased number of partitions, decreased phase encoding steps, or rectangular field of view. Widening bandwidth also makes the scan faster but at the expense of a significant reduction of signal-to-noise ratio.

Thoracic 3D MRA can be obtained in different orientations such as sagittal, coronal or sagittal oblique directions that are most suitable for visualization of the target vascular structure. For the visualization of pulmonary arteries, for example, 3D MRA should be performed in the coronal plane for both lungs and the sagittal plane for just one lung. For optimal diagnostic evaluation of the thoracic aorta and subclavian arteries a coronal acquisition is usually recommended. However, sagittal oblique imaging planes are recommended for higher resolution images of the aortic arch optimizing anatomic coverage using the highest possible spatial resolution (i.e., smallest voxel size) (Fig. **1.17**). Sagittal acquisitions also have the advantage of facilitating the use of fractional or rectangular fields of view with minimal concerns from aliasing (wrapping) of the image data. A rectangular field of view shortens the overall scan time, thereby reducing the breath-holding time.

Gadolinium contrast media are typically administered intravenously via an MR-compatible injector or via hand injection when power injectors are unavailable or cannot be used. The contrast bolus should always be followed by adequate saline flush (typically 15–20 ml) to ensure that the entire contrast media bolus has been

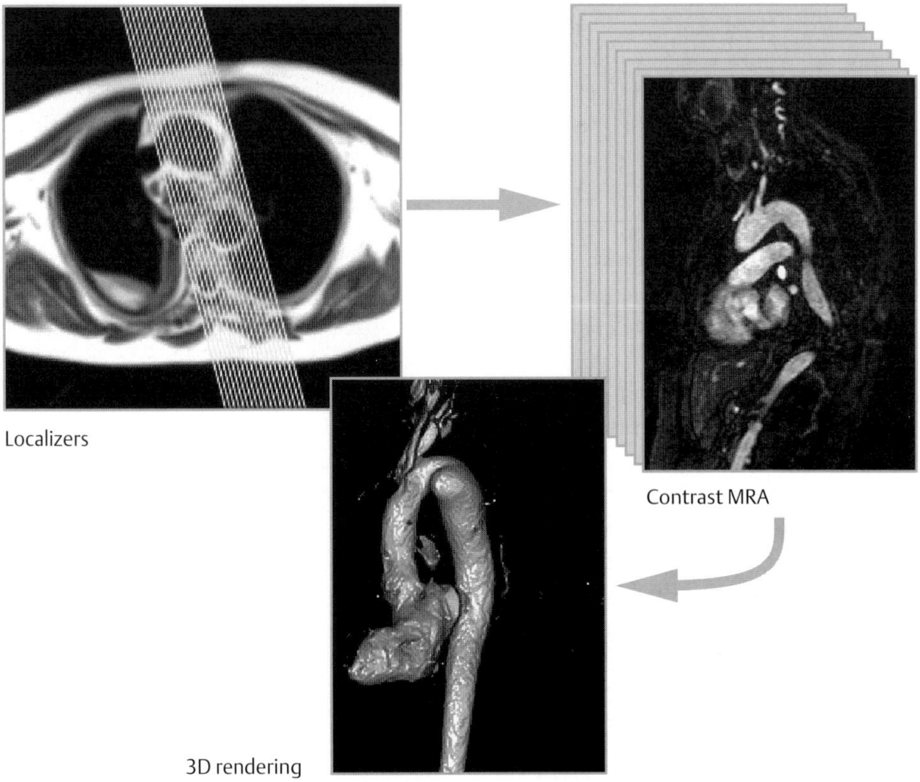

Fig. 1.**17** Contrast-enhanced MR angiography images obtained in contiguous adjacent planes, and the resulting 3D-shaded surface-rendered image.

administered at the proper rate. The right arm is the preferred intravenous site because it has a more direct path to the heart compared to the left arm. Earlier studies have shown that a gadolinium dose of 0.2 mmol/kg (roughly between 20 to 40 ml) injected at a rate of 2 ml/sec is optimal for imaging large thoracic vessels. A weight-dependent dose is also applicable to pediatric cases [23] provided that the contrast bolus could be diluted for volumes lower that 5 ml to maintain a minimum injection volume of 5 ml (see Table 1.**1**).

Table 1.1 Calculated doses of gadolinium for contrast-enhanced angiograms of the heart and thoracic vessels for ranges of pediatric and adult body weights. Notice that for pediatric doses below 5 ml we suggest that the contrast media might be diluted in saline to maintain a minimum bolus volume of 5 ml.

MAGNEVIST (Gd-DTPA; 0.5 molar)					1 ml = 0.5 mmol
Pediatric doses		0.3 mmol/kg 0.6 ml/kg	**Adult doses**		0.2 mmol/kg 0.4 ml/kg
Body Weight		Volume	Body Weight		Volume
kg	lb	mL	kg	lb	mL
2	4	3*	40	88	16
3	7	3*	42	92	17
4	9	3*	44	97	18
5	11	3	46	101	18
6	13	4	48	106	19
7	15	4	50	110	20
8	18	5	52	114	21
9	20	5	54	119	22
10	22	6	56	123	22
11	24	7	58	128	23
12	26	7	60	132	24
13	29	8	62	136	25
14	31	8	64	141	26
15	33	9	66	145	26
16	35	10	68	150	27
17	37	10	70	154	28
18	40	11	72	158	29
19	42	11	74	163	30
20	44	12	76	167	30
21	46	13	78	172	31
22	48	13	80	176	32
23	51	14	82	180	33
24	53	14	84	185	34
25	55	15	86	189	34
26	57	16	88	194	35
27	59	16	90	198	36
28	62	17	92	202	37
29	64	17	94	207	38
30	66	18	96	211	38
31	68	19	98	216	39
32	70	19	100	220	40
33	73	20	102	224	40*
34	75	20	104	229	40*
35	77	21	106	233	40*
36	79	22	108	238	40*
37	81	22	110	242	40*
38	84	23	112	246	40*
39	86	23	114	251	40*

*Volumes listed do not include bolus used for timing the transit time
*Volumes below 5 ml might be deluted 1:1 with saline
*Contrast injection must be followed by saline injection of:
 ~ at least 10 ml of saline for pediatric patients
 ~ at least 20 ml of saline for adult patients

1.2.10 Flow Quantification and Velocity-Encoded Cine Sequences

Use of phase-contrast (PC) imaging techniques with gradient motion rephasing (GMR) results in different phases of moving voxels in a given plane compared to stationary voxels. The application of short-lived magnetic gradients allows each point in the imaging plane to be encoded with a phase shift that is directly proportional to the velocity at that point. The resulting images, called phase-contrast (PC) images or velocity-encoded cine images (VEC), provide a topographic map of instantaneous velocities of each pixel in the image. A pulse sequence for velocity mapping can be designed to gave the velocity-encoding within or through the imaging plane as well as in all three directions. The in-plane technique has been used mainly to measure flow velocities, and the advantage of the technique is that the velocity distribution along, for example, a stenotic jet can be displayed in the velocity map, which enables determination of the peak velocity. Partial volume effects may arise during in-plane examinations of narrow stenotic jets. The through-plane technique is less sensitive to these effects, but the drawback of this technique of measuring the stenotic peak velocity is that the exact location may not be predicted in advance. The major advantage of the through-plane technique, however, is the ability to measure volume flow as the product of the cross-sectional area and the average velocity within a region-of-interest (ROI). By integrating the flow volume for all images during the cardiac cycle it is possible to calculate the total volume ejected during a single heart beat. This technique is commonly used for quantification of right ventricular (RV) and left ventricular (LV) outputs and the quantitative assessment of cardiac shunts (Fig. **1.18**). The same technique is also used to evaluate forward and regurgitant flows across the aortic or pulmonary valve and evaluate the degree of valvular insufficiency from the regurgitant fraction. Similarly, velocity-encoded images can be used to establish an accurate peak velocity across a stenotic valve to quantify the severity of the stenosis. An approximation of the pressure gradient across the valve can also be obtained from the modified Bernoulli equation. This technique is very similar to the one used in Doppler echocardiography [24]. One of the critical source of errors is the misalignment between the imaging plane and the direction of the flow. Misalignment between the direction of flow and the direction of the motion-encoding magnetic gradients can be avoided in the through-plane technique by careful angulation of the imaging plane perpendicular to the flow direction. In the absence of partial volume errors, a misalignment of as much as 20° will produce only a 6% error, whereas a more realistic misalignment of 5° causes an error of < 1% [61]. Under ideal conditions, the volume flow in a vessel can be quantified from a through-plane velocity map as the average velocity within an ROI multiplied by the cross-sectional area of the ROI. However, a general problem is the size of the chosen ROI. If the ROI is smaller than the cross-section of the vessel, then the volume flow is underestimated. On the other hand, random errors are related to an ROI much larger than the lumen of the vessel, because the flow-related phase shift will vanish within the noise from the stationary tissue due to a limited signal-to-noise ratio. Another source of errors and erroneous mea-

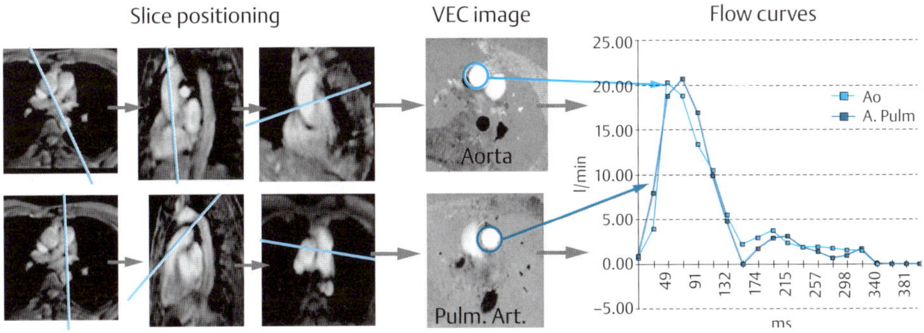

Fig. 1.**18** Example of quantitative analysis of aortic blood flow using velocity-encoded cine (VEC) phase contrast images. The imaging plane is carefully positioned perpendicular to the vessel and the blood flow curves are calculated from a region of interest assigned over the VEC images. The curves of aortic and pulmonary flow in a normal subject are shown here.

surements comes from the fact that phase is cyclic, giving a natural limit of $\pm\pi$ radians to the maximum angular range that can be measured without phase wrap and ambiguity of the velocity data. Thus, the predicted peak velocity should cover approximately two-thirds of the available phase interval to avoid aliasing of the velocity data while retaining adequate sensitivity.

1.3 Post-Processing and Rendering Techniques

1.3.1 Multiplanar Reformatting (MPR)

The acquisition of 3D data in contiguous volume slabs allows for images to be resampled or reformatted in an oblique orientation. From the 3D data set of MR angiography data, for example, it is possible to obtain 2D images in any oblique plane across the volume of data. Traditionally, the standard viewing and processing software programs allow automatic reformatting of the data in orthogonal planes, such as coronal and sagittal planes, that can be calculated from transverse axial planes. More advanced post-processing algorithms allow the users to easily “navigate” through a volume of 3D data by interactively positioning an oblique plane across the data and selecting the most appropriate angle for viewing a specific anatomic feature. This is particularly useful in cardiovascular imaging where most of the anatomic structures are seldom aligned with the standard orthogonal planes of the human body. In many instances it is necessary to apply multiple oblique tilts to the image plane to align it to a vessel or a cardiac structure that needs to be visualized (Fig. 1.**19**). This is even more critical when quantitative measurements are applied such as when measurements of vessel diameters are extracted from the images. In this particular case it is necessary to align the image plane with the central axis of the vessel to avoid measurement

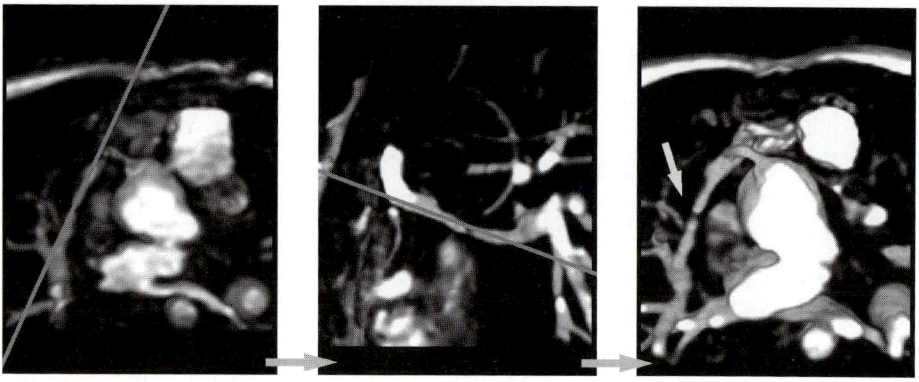

Fig. 1.**19** Example of "oblique" MPR images obtained from a set of 3D volume contrast-enhanced MR angiogram images. Oblique planes are reconstructed along a pulmonary vessel to better visualize a segmental stenosis.

errors from oblique slicing or partial volume of the vessel being falsely measured as the true diameter of the vessel.

The unique ability to resample 3D data in any oblique plane is one of the most valuable features of MR cardiovascular imaging techniques that is far superior to the other imaging modalities such as echocardiography and X-ray angiography that rely essentially on adequate plane positioning during the acquisition of the study and lack the flexibility of viewing the data in different orientation a posteriori. Also the ability of MRI to acquire true 3D volumes with matched resolution in the 3 spatial directions is unique while other tomographic imaging techniques such as computed tomography require very fast and very high resolution acquisition devices to generate similar types of volumetric data.

1.3.2 "Thick-Slab" MPR

With high target-to-background contrast images such as those of MR angiography it is often desirable to vary the slice thickness to obtain 2D reformatted images from 3D data sets that contain the required anatomic structures. This is particularly true for angiographic data where, by increasing the thickness of the reconstructed orthogonal or oblique plane, one gets a better view of multiple vessel branches and ramifications. Sophisticated rendering techniques allow one to select the best rendering parameters for these "thick-slab" images. Most commonly the rendering technique is either a maximum intensity projection (see next section for details) or a volume/surface rendering combination that will optimally provide a realistic view of the data and give a better depth perception of the different vascular structures (see Fig. 1.**20**).

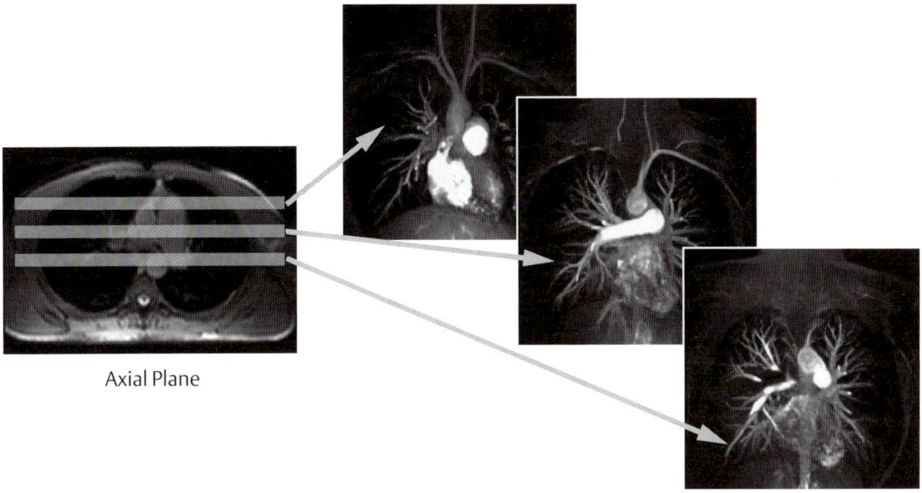

Fig. 1.**20** Example of "thick-slab" MPR images obtained from a set of 3D volume contrast-enhanced MR angiogram images of the thoracic vessels.

1.3.3 Curved-Oblique Reformatted Images

Because most vascular structures follow curved and tortuous paths, it is often very difficult to find a proper oblique orientation of a single plane that will show the complete vascular segment. Although 3D rendering techniques will allow visualization of the path of a given vessel, it is often desirable to "flatten" the vessel on a single plane to better assess anatomic shapes and dimensions of that vessel or of a given tortuous anatomic structure. Computer-generated images can be obtained from a manually drawn curved path across the 3D data set. This is particularly useful for visualizing and measuring dimensions and shapes of tortuous vessels such as an aortic arch that cannot be evaluated in a single 2D plane (see Fig. 1.**21**).

In addition to the ability of reformatting 3D data sets into 2D image planes, there are a variety of computer-generated rendering techniques that can be applied to cardiovascular MRA. The tremendous advancements in computer graphic and 3D rendering techniques from the entertainment and graphic industry have benefited the medical imaging arena as well. Powerful software and hardware engines allow for real-time 3D rendering of large data sets that can be interactively manipulated to obtain the best possible view of a given anatomic structure. In most cases the users will have a variety of rendering options to choose from and an overwhelming number of rendering parameters that can be adjusted to achieve different visual and rendering effects. The selection of the optimal rendering techniques with the most appropriate parameters will often vary depending on the type of anatomic structure that is being

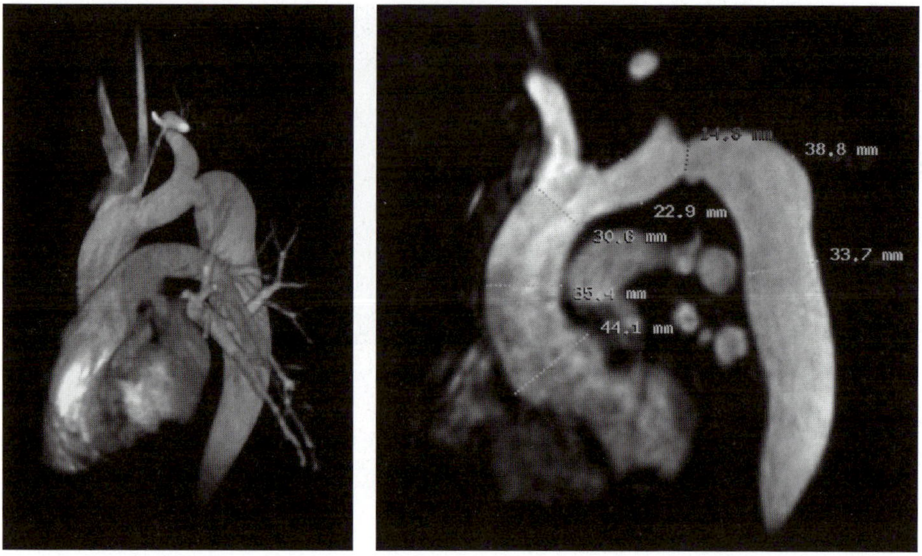

A 3D MRA B "curved" reformatted image

Fig. 1.**21** Example of curved-reformatting of a tortuous aortic arch where the resulting image is a reconstructed plane along the center line of the aorta that allows the visualization and measurement of the real middle diameter of the vessel.

evaluated and on the clinical question being addressed. Different rendering techniques will be used, for example, if the topological relationship of different organs is being addressed or if a particular shape and morphology of a given structure is being evaluated. A brief description of some of the basic rendering techniques is described in the following sections.

1.3.4 Maximum Intensity Projections (MIP)

The maximum intensity projection technique (MIP) is the simplest and most widely used technique for visualization of 3D MR angiography data. It is based on a simple algorithm of projecting all the data on to one plane by selecting the highest intensity data element (voxel) in the data set along the projection lines. The resulting image is similar to angiographic images obtained from traditional X-ray angiography. This technique is only applicable to high target-to-background contrast images with limited amount of anatomic structures. Because it does not differentiate front from back, adjacent structures will overlap resulting in a difficult visual appreciation of the true spatial location of a given structure. Because MIP projections can be generated from any viewing angle it is often necessary to generate multiple MIP views from different view angles around the vascular structure of interest. By dynamically reviewing the

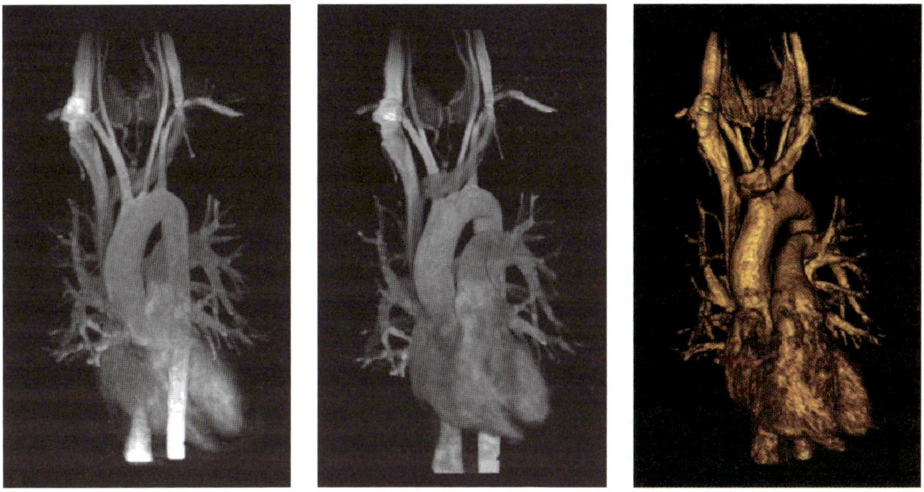

A MIP (Maximum Intensity Projection) **B** Volume Rendering (Depth encoding) **C** Surface Rendering (Shaded surfaces)

Fig. 1.**22** Example of different 3D rendering techniques of contrast-enhanced MRA. From left to right: maximum intensity projection (MIP), depth-encoded volume rendering, and opaque surface rendering.

images obtained from these different angles in a pseudo-movie mode, it is often easier for the human eye to perceive the true three-dimensional location of the different anatomic structure. Static MIP images are often much more difficult to interpret especially, if multiple vascular structures overlap. MIP is particularly convenient for peripheral vascular structures where there is a limited number of vessels and very minimal spatial overlap. It has the advantage that it does not require any thresholding that would eliminate small and low contrast vessels, but it projects all the data available in the 3D data set and the user can still apply window and level adjustments to obtain the best contrast for the desired vascular structure. MIP does not apply very well for central and large structures such as the heart and great vessels of the mediastinal area where multiple adjacent structures overlap and prevent adequate visualization of individual anatomic structures.

1.3.5 Surface Rendering and Volume Rendering

Because the MIP rendering technique is suboptimal for visualizing large overlapping structures, it is often necessary to apply alternative rendering techniques that will introduce a certain degree of opacity that will allow one to better perceive the anatomic structures proximal to the viewing points and occlude structures that are located behind them (Fig. 1.**22**). The typical "shaded surface" rendering technique is based on a completely different algorithm called "ray-tracing", a technique commonly used in computer animation applications. The surface rendering technique requires the exact identification of a surface or “threshold” between the object of interest and the surrounding structures. The selected object must be identified either by manual or automatic contouring techniques or by simple thresholding techniques, taking advantage of the high contrast of the vascular structures in comparison with the surrounding anatomic structures. Once the contours of the object have been identified, the computer algorithm will apply pseudo-realistic rendering techniques to the surface of that object with parameters such as light, shadows, color and texture. Computer graphics techniques have made such tremendous progress in the last few years that it is possible today to apply very sophisticated rendering algorithms that provide very realistic views of the organ or anatomic structure being evaluated. Interactive adjustment of lighting conditions, texture and reflection parameters of the surface of the 3D object can enhance the visual perception of complex anatomic structures.

The main limitation of the surface rendering technique is that it relies on the arbitrary selection of a given boundary between the object of interest and the surrounding structures. In the case of angiographic data this requires adequate delineation of the vascular anatomy. Because most segmentation algorithms will rely on difference in intensity between the opacified vessel and the surrounding tissue, they will often eliminate vascular structures and small vessels that have low contrast intensity. Also, the exact delineation of the vessels may vary significantly depending on the threshold used for setting an arbitrary boundary between the vessel and surrounding structure. A threshold set too high will make the vessel appear narrower than reality and a threshold set too high will include low contrast structures surrounding the vessels that will occlude and alter the true shape of the vascular tree.

More advanced rendering techniques nowadays rely on sophisticated combinations of transparency and opacity of different anatomic structures. Under the common denomination of “volume rendering” there are a variety of sophisticated rendering algorithms that will assign different degrees of opacity and even different colors and textures to objects in the volume of interest. Volume rendering techniques still rely on the selection of a range of intensity values to identify the anatomic structures, but they do not necessarily require an exact border or outline of an object, and will account for progressive changes in intensity around the edges. Furthermore, by applying different transparency factors, it is possible to show the low intensity and smaller structures that have a lower contrast ratio (Fig. 1.**23**).

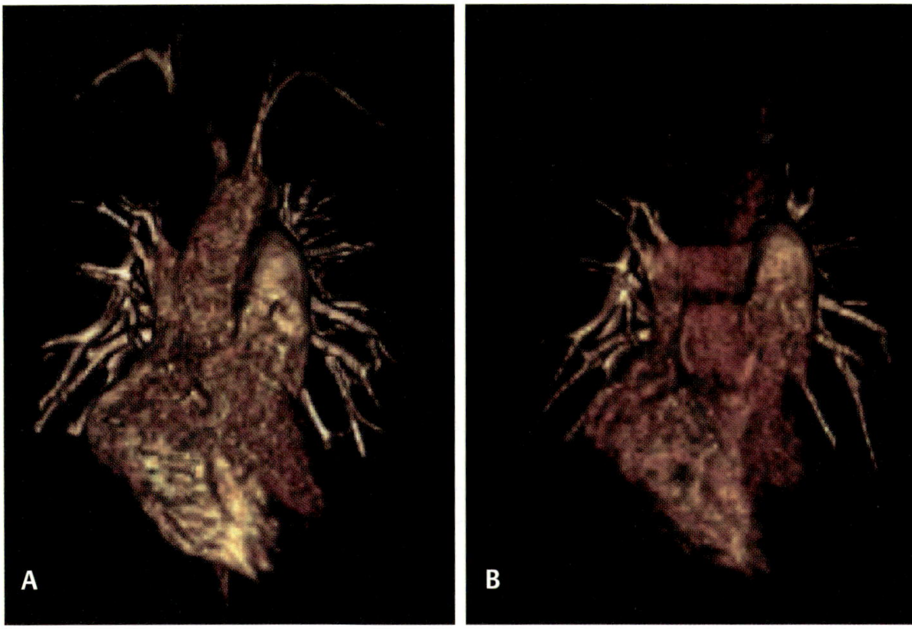

Fig. 1.**23** Example of different volume rendering settings with different opacities. The image on the right with partial transparency allows better visualization of the right pulmonary artery behind the ascending aorta.

1.4 References

1. Higgins CB. Overview of MR of the heart. AJR 1986; 146: 907–918.
2. Boxt LM. Cardiac MR imaging: A guide for the beginner. RadioGraphics 1999; 19: 1009–1025.
3. Didier D, Ratib O, Friedli B, et al. Cine gradient-echo MR imaging in the evaluation of cardiovascular disease. RadioGraphics 1993; 13: 561–573.
4. Garcia E, Bonow RO, Richie JL, et al. Standardization of cardiac tomographic imaging. J Nucl Med 1992; 33: 1434–1435.
5. Ratib O, Didier D, Chatelain P, Righetti A, Lerch R, Townsend D. Standard views in cardiac multimodality tomographic imaging. Am J Card Im 1995; 9: 67–76.
6. Bloomgarden DC, Fayad ZA, Ferrari VA, Chin B, Sutton MG, Axel L. Global cardiac function using fast breath-hold MRI: validation of new acquisition and analysis techniques. Magn Reson Med 1997; 37: 683–692.
7. Sakuma H, Globits S, Bourne MW, Shimakawa A, Foo TK, Higgins CB. Improved reproducibility in measuring LV volumes and mass using multicoil breath-hold cine MR imaging. J Magn Reson Imaging 19566; 6: 124–127.
8. Lanzer P, Barta C, Bovinick EH, et al. ECG-synchronized cardiac MR imaging: method and evaluation. Radiology 1985; 155: 681–686.

9. Van Genderingen HR, Sprenger M, De Ridder JW, Van Rossum AC. Carbon-fiber electrodes and leads for electrocardiography during MR imaging. Radiology 1989; 171: 852.
10. Pirolo JS, Branham BH, Creswell LL, Perman WH, Vannier MW, Pasque MK. Pressure-gated acquisition of cardiac MR images. Radiology 1992; 183: 487–492.
11. Atkinson DJ, Edelman RR. Cine-angiography of the heart in a single breath hold with a segmented turbo-FLASH sequence. Radiology 1991; 178: 357–360.
12. Davis CP, McKinnon GC, Debatin JF, Duewell S, von Schulthess G. Single-shot versus interleaved echoplanar MR imaging: application to visualization of cardiac valve leaflets. J Magn Reson Imaging 1995; 5: 107–112.
13. Pereles FS, Kapoor V, Carr JC, Simonetti OP, Krupinski EA, Baskaran V, Finn JP. Usefulness of segmented true-FISP cardiac pulse sequence in evaluation of congenital and acquired adult cardiac abnormalities AJR 2001; 177: 1155–1160.
14. Atkinson D, Teresi L. Magnetic resonance angiography. Magn Reson Q 1994; 10: 149–172.
15. Hany TF, McKinnon GC, Lueng DA, Pfannater T, Debatin JF. Optimization of contrast timing for breath-hold three dimensional MR angiography. J Magn Reson Imaging 1997; 7: 551–556.
16. Neimatallah MA, Ho VB, Dong Q, Williams D, Patel S, Song JH, Prince M. Gadolinium-enhanced 3D magnetic resonance angiography of the thoracic vessels. J Magn Res Imaging 1999; 10: 758–770.
17. Leung DA, Debatin JF. Three-dimensional contrast-enhanced magnetic resonance angiography of the thoracic vasculature. Eur Radiol 1997; 7: 981–989.
18. Krinsky GA, Rofsky N, Flyer M, et al. Thoracic aorta: comparison of gadolinium-enhanced three-dimensional MR angiography with conventional MR imaging. Radiology 1007; 202: 183–193.
19. Prince MR, Chenevert TL, Foo TKF, Londy FJ, Ward JS, Maki JH. Contrast-enhanced abdominal MR angiography: Optimization of imaging delay time by automating the detection of contrast material arrival in the aorta. Radiology 1997; 203: 109–114.
20. Earls JP, Rofsky NM, DeCorato DR, Krinsky GA, Weinreb JC. Breath-hold single-dose gadolinium-enhanced three-dimensional MR aortography: Usefulness of a timing examination and MR power injrector. Radiology 1996; 201: 705–710.
21. Foo TKF, Saranathan M, Prince MR, Chenevert TL. Automated detection of bolus arrival and initiation of data acquisition in fast gadolinium-enhanced MR angiography. Radiology 1997; 203: 275–280.
22. Kim JK, Farb RI, Wright GA. Test bolus examination in the carotid artery at dynamic gadolinium-enhanced MR angiography. Radiology 1998; 206: 283–289.
23. Wai-man Lam W, Chan JHM, Hui Y, Chan FL. Non-breath-hold gadolinium-enhanced MR angiography of the thoracoabdominal aorta: experience in 18 children. AJR 1998; 170: 478–480.
24. Lee VS, Spritzer CE, Carroll BA, et al. Flow quantification using fast cine phase-contrast MR imaging, conventional cine phase-contrast MR imaging, and Doppler sonography: in vitro and in vivo validation. Am J Roentgenol 1997; 169: 1125–1131.

2 Congenital Heart Disease

Magnetic resonance imaging (MRI) is a well-established complementary technique to echocardiography equal or even superior to other imaging modalities in the preoperative and postoperative assessment of congenital heart disease (CHD) [1–4]. The ability of this non-invasive technique to depict anatomic and morphological anomalies, assess cardiac function and quantitatively evaluate hemodynamic alterations has increased its role in diagnostic imaging processes [5,6]. MRI is particularly useful in cases where echocardiography is limited, such as in the assessment of great arteries and veins of the thorax [7,8], investigation of complex anomalies and the follow-up of surgical repairs [9]. With the development of advanced cardiovascular surgery for complex CHD, an increasing number of patients (with palliative procedures or complete repair) requires numerous follow-up examinations and MRI is often the procedure of choice for detecting residual defects or surgical complications [10,11,12].

Cardiac MRI techniques are in constant evolution and new imaging techniques are being developed, such as fast gradient-echo (GE) sequences, flow-sensitive MRI technique [13–17] and MR angiography [18,19], providing better and more widely adopted imaging techniques for preoperative evaluation of some CHD. MR study is not limited to morphologic evaluation provided by the spin-echo technique but in the majority of cases is complemented by functional data and flow measurements in a single examination. Velocity-encoded cine sequences (VEC) provide more accurate and more reproducible information for quantifying non-invasively valvular regurgitation after surgical repair and for evaluating valvular or vascular stenosis in areas of limited echocardiographic access [20]. It can also be used for non-invasive quantification of cardiac shunts and separate measurement of right and left pulmonary flows. Furthermore, cine-GE MRI allows quantitative ventricular function measurement (particularly the right ventricular function), which is ideally suitable for long-term follow-up as well as for preoperative evaluation of patients with CHD for identifying the optimal timing for surgical interventions.

This chapter describes the role of the different types of MR imaging techniques in the pre- and postoperative evaluation of CHD with emphasis on the segmental approach of these anomalies. For dynamic images of selected CHD cases, see the first and second chapters on the companion CD-ROM.

2.1 Major Indications of MRI in CHD

The clinical role of MRI in the evaluation of patients with CHD is now well established and has been reported and recommended by the Task Force of the European Society of

Cardiology [21]. MRI is particularly suitable for the assessment of supracardiac structures and in general in older children and adults and in cases of complex anatomy.

The major clinical indications of MRI are:

1. Segmental description of cardiac anomalies.
2. Evaluation of thoracic aortic anomalies.
3. Evaluation of cono-truncal malformations and complex anomalies.
4. Identification of pulmonary and systemic venous anomalies.
5. Non-invasive detection and quantification of shunts, stenoses and regurgitations.
6. Post-operative studies and evaluation of CHD in adult patients.

2.2 Imaging Techniques

2.2.1 Sedation, Monitoring and Patient Preparation

Children younger than 6 years of age undergoing a cardiac MRI procedure should be sedated. Sedation is usually not necessary for older children, provided that prior explanation of the procedure is given to the patient in the presence of the parents that can help to reassure and calm the child. Oral sedation using chloral hydrate (50–100 mg/kg) or pentobarbital administered intramuscularly (5–6 mg/kg) are commonly used. The availability of an anesthesiologist in the MR unit offers the possibility to use propofol (Diprivan) in continuous perfusion, allowing rapid and deep sedation with rapid recovery. Short periods of apnea are also possible with an additional dose administered in bolus, without need to intubate the patient, allowing the use of breath-hold MR angiographic techniques, thus improving significantly the quality of images. ECG signal, oxygen saturation will be monitored with the help of an MR compatible system. Small children will be examined within a head coil whereas for older patients the best results will be obtained by using a specific cardiac coil or a flexible thoracic or abdominal coil.

2.2.2 Spin-Echo Technique

The ECG-gated spin-echo multislice technique remains the basic, most commonly used technique for the depiction of abnormal morphology in CHD [22,23]. An odd firing order of the slices allows the first slice of the series (which can be subject to artifacts because it occurs during the isovolumetric contraction phase and because of entry slice phenomenon) to be away from the region of interest. Contiguous slices are acquired in 6 to 10 minutes with a slice thickness according to patient heart size and varying from 3 to 10 mm. Presaturation slabs above and below the slices may help to reduce flow artifacts, particularly in venous structures but it also reduces the total number of slices. Transverse images will be first carried out encompassing the great vessels and the entire heart. Then, one or two additional planes will be acquired, particularly in complex diseases: coronal and sagittal oblique in the plane of the

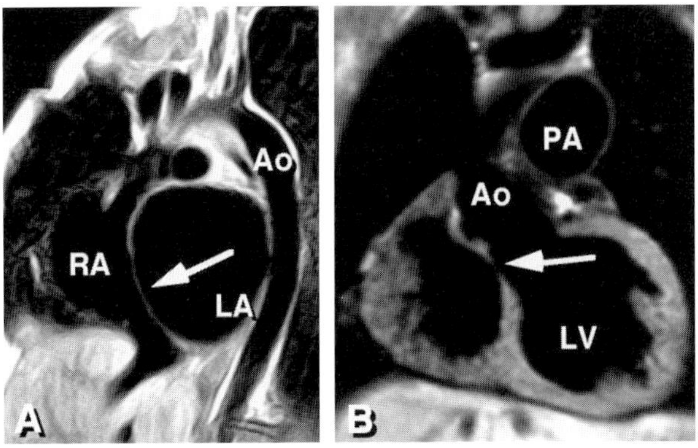

Fig. 2.1 Sagittal (**A**) and coronal (**B**) spin-echo images using a large matrix (256 × 512) allow one to visualize very thin structures such as fossa ovalis (**A**) and membranous septum (**B**) (arrows), the most frequent sites of atrial septal and ventricular septal defects. Ao = aorta, PA = pulmonary artery, LV = left ventricle, RA = right atrium, LA = left atrium.

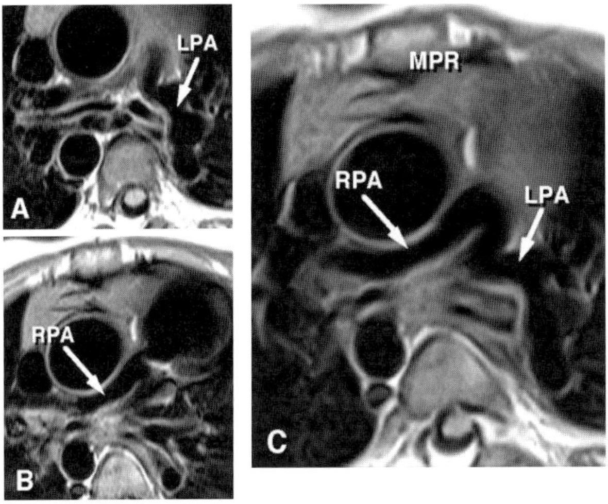

Fig. 2.2 Transverse spin-echo images in a case of pulmonary atresia after pulmonary valvotomy. Pulmonary bifurcation cannot be depicted on one plane because of the oblique course of the right and left pulmonary branches (**A**, **B**). By using the same curved multiplanar reconstruction technique as in MR angiography, the pulmonary confluence can be demonstrated (**C**). RPA = right pulmonary artery, LPA = left pulmonary artery.

thoracic aorta or the true short axis of the heart determined on the transverse images, depending on the abnormalities encountered. For these two additional planes one can use a fast spin-echo sequence with an echo train of 2 which allows a reduction of the acquisition time by a factor of 2. In this technique, the total number of slices will be reduced. Thus, it will not be recommended for transverse images but for other planes where fewer images are necessary. Because the first purpose of imaging in congenital anomalies is the depiction of morphology, one can improve spatial resolution by using a large matrix of up to 256 × 512 pixels in the read direction which allows one to visualize very thin anatomic structures such as the fossa ovalis and membranous septum (Fig. 2.1) The quality of the images is also improved when using two or three signal averages. In some cases where the anatomic structure is not depicted on one plane because of oblique or tortuous course, a multiplanar reconstruction technique can also be applied to help identify the abnormal morphology of some crucial structures (Fig. 2.2).

2.2.3 Cine-MR Imaging

Cine-MR imaging is commonly obtained using gradient-echo (GE) pulse sequences at multiple phases of the cardiac cycle with typical TR equal to 20 to 30 milliseconds, TE equal to 5 to 12 milliseconds and a flip angle of 30 degrees requiring as little as 2 to 5 minutes of acquisition time. Usually, 16 frames are sufficient to cover the cardiac cycle and are displayed in a cine loop allowing a dynamic approach. These cine-GE sequences are particularly suitable for evaluating cardiac function [24,25]. Abnormal flow encountered in the cardiac chambers and great vessels are detectable by this technique appearing as signal voids due to turbulence and acceleration of flow within normally high signal intensity of the blood pool [26,27]. It has been demonstrated previously that the extent and contrast of the signal void is dependent upon technical factors, particularly the TE and tends to decrease when using short TE [28]. This fact must be kept in mind when evaluating flow anomalies encountered in CHD (shunts, stenotic lesion or valvular regurgitation) (see Chapter 5 on valvular heart diseases and the fourth chapter on the CD-ROM).

One way to decrease the acquisition time considerably when using cine-GE technique is to use k space segmentation. This technique (phase encoding grouping) allows one to reduce the imaging time by a factor of 2 or 3 depending upon the heart rate while keeping a correct spatial resolution with a matrix such as 256 × 256. Thus, one can continue using long TE sequences for evaluating abnormal flow patterns, avoiding too long acquisition times.

Fast GE sequences with typical TR value of 4 to 8 milliseconds and TE equal to 2 to 4 milliseconds have recently been used, allowing cine-images to be acquired within a single breath-hold, thus eliminating respiratory artifacts. These sequences are ideal to evaluate cardiac function [29]. In CHD, it is important to evaluate not only left ventricular function as in the majority of the cases in adult cardiology but also the right ventricular function, which is one of the major limitations of echocardiography. For the evaluation of thoracic aorta and aortic arch diseases, particularly in cases with tortuous vessel, multiple cine sequences acquired in adjacent planes with partial overlap can be subsequently rendered using the maximum intensity projection algorithm (MIP). The resulting image corresponding to the sum of the adjacent planes can be shown in a cine loop as a standard cine, showing the entire thickness of the vessel and adding a volume effect while maintaining the flow information provided by the cine sequences (see Chapter 3 and the second chapter of the CD-ROM).

2.2.4 Flow-Sensitive Imaging Techniques

The most popular flow-sensitive cine-MR technique used today is the phase change technique based on the principle that the phase of flowing spins relative to stationary spins along a magnetic gradient changes in direct proportion to the velocity of flow. This technique, also called velocity-encoded cine-MR imaging (VEC-MRI) allows quantification of blood flow velocity and volume flow in cardiac chambers and great vessels [30–33]. The VEC-MRI technique is based upon the acquisition of two sets of images, usually acquired simultaneously: one with and one without velocity encoding. The subtraction of the two images allows the calculation of a phase shift that is proportional to the velocity of flow along the direction of the flow compensation gradient. Images can be reconstructed in magnitude, providing anatomic information and in phase, providing flow velocity information. The phase shift, proportional to the velocity, is displayed as variations in pixel intensity on the phase map image. On this image, stationary tissue appears in gray whereas flow in the positive or negative direction along the flow-encoding axis will appear as bright or dark pixels, respectively. Thus, one can differentiate antegrade from retrograde flow [34]. Velocity can be encoded either on planes perpendicular to the direction of flow by using slice-selective direction (through-plane velocity measurement) or parallel to the direction of flow by using phased-encoded or frequency-encoded directions (in-plane velocity measurement) or simultaneously in three orthogonal dimensions [34].

VEC-MRI can be used to calculate the absolute blood velocity at each point in the cardiac cycle in a given location. The velocity can be measured for each pixel or within a region of interest (ROI) around the entire area or parts of a vessel cross-section or across a valve annulus. Based on the measurement of the cross-sectional area of a vascular lumen or a valve annulus on the magnitude image, the product of area and mean velocity (average value for all pixels in the cross-sectional area on the phase image) yields the instantaneous flow volume for a specific time frame in the cardiac cycle. Integration of all instantaneous flow volumes throughout the cardiac cycle gives the volume flow per heartbeat. This technique has been evaluated in vitro as well as in vivo by several authors to yield accurate measurements of aortic and pulmonary artery flows, representing the stroke volumes of the left ventricle and the right ventricle, respectively [24]. It has been used as well in the calculation of pulmonary-to-systemic flow ratio so allowing non-invasive quantification of left-to-right shunts [35,36], separate measurement of right and left pulmonary flows [37] and quantitative assessment of valvular regurgitation [6].

For quantification of a stenotic lesion, VEC-MR allows one to measure directly the increase of flow velocity in the jet of blood passing though the stenosis [5,38]. The calculation of the peak velocity or maximum velocity (V_{max}) within the stenotic jet can be carried out either on planes perpendicular to the direction of flow (through-plane velocity measurement) or parallel to the direction of flow (in-plane velocity measurement). In-plane imaging yields numerous pixels for analysis of velocity because the entire abnormal jet is displayed. But in the case of a very tight stenosis, where the jet is narrowed, in-plane measurement may be less reliable because of partial volume averaging and motion of the jet out of the imaging plane. Conversely, with through-plane imaging, only a slice of the jet is displayed and one can miss the maximum velocity if the plane is too far from the origin of the stenosis. On the other hand, misregistration of flow due to signal loss depending upon turbulence and eddy currents may occur if the plane is too close to the origin of the stenosis. Thus, it is preferable to measure data in both in- and through-planes [34]. The calculation of

V_{max} is usually easy for velocities less than 4 m/sec but for velocities up to 6 m/sec the use of short TE sequence (TE = 3–4 ms) is mandatory to improve the reliability and accuracy of the measurements [39]. The pressure gradient (ΔP) across a stenotic valve can be derived using the modified Bernoulli equation:

$$\Delta P = 4 \cdot (V_{max})^2$$

where ΔP is the pressure drop across the stenosis and V_{max} the peak velocity in m/sec measured within the stenotic jet.

2.2.5 Gadolinium-Enhanced 3D MR Angiography

Three-dimensional (3D) gadolinium-enhanced MR angiography has been recommended by several authors for evaluating thoracic vessels after it was demonstrated to be particularly useful in the diagnosis and assessment of congenital anomalies [18,19]. Initial studies were made by using non-breath-hold techniques, which provided high-quality projections, but respiratory motion degrades the quality of images of the intrathoracic great vessels. Recently, the use of breath-hold techniques with short TR and TE allows one to minimize respiration-induced motion artifacts and reduce acquisition time. These MR angiography techniques provide cross-sectional data including intraluminal as well as extraluminal components of the vascular disease, thus yielding a unique information. The images obtained by these techniques are usually processed on a computer workstation and can be further reconstructed using different rendering and reformatting techniques, such as the maximum intensity projection (MIP) algorithm which provides images similar to conventional contrast X-ray angiography. However, this reconstruction technique has limitations such as overestimation of vascular stenoses. In some cases, the original images can be first segmented to remove superimpositions of undesirable overlapping vascular and anatomic structures and to minimize wrap-around artifacts (aliasing).

Other image reconstruction and rendering techniques include thick-slice multiplanar reformation (MPR) and 3D surface rendering (SR) or volume rendering (VR) (see Chapter 1 and 3 of this book and chapter 2 of the companion CD-ROM).

2.3 Segmental Description of Cardiac Anomalies

The first step in the diagnostics of CHD with any imaging modality is to analyze the heart segment by segment and the more complex the congenital abnormality, the more necessary is this sequential approach [40,41]. Thus, when interpreting MR images, the description will comprise the definition of the atrial situs, the type of ventricular loop, the type of cono-truncus and position of the great vessels and finally, the intersegmental connections.

For determination of the atrial situs, the best anatomic method is to define the morphology of the appendages. The right atrial appendage is triangular and broad-based whereas the left atrial appendage has a tubular configuration and its atrial junction is narrowed. In practice, this method remains difficult, even with a multiplanar technique such as MRI. The morphology and position of the abdominal viscera (liver, spleen and stomach) and the position and relationship of the aorta and inferior vena cava is the second way to determine the atrial situs. But this can be difficult when there is an interruption of the inferior vena cava and azygos continuation. Thus, the best way to determine the atrial situs is the morphology and relationship of the main bronchi and pulmonary arteries. MRI is the only method that shows both structures in different planes. This relationship will be established on transverse and coronal images. The morphologically right main bronchus is short and vertical, whereas the morphologically left main bronchus is longer and more horizontal. The right pulmonary artery courses anterior then lateral to the right bronchus whereas the left pulmonary artery courses over the left bronchus. This relationship defines the atrial situs solitus. If the morphologically left bronchus and left pulmonary artery are right-sided, this indicates atrial situs inversus. If the bronchi and the pulmonary arteries show similar morphology, this indicates atrial situs ambiguous. Bilateral right main bronchi and right pulmonary arteries suggest right-sided isomerism (often associated with asplenia) whereas bilateral left main bronchi and left pulmonary arteries indicate left-sided isomerism (frequently encountered with polysplenia and azygos vein continuation) (Fig. 2.**3**).

Determination of the ventricular loop will be easily possible on transverse images. Each ventricle will be identified by its own morphology and by its atrioventricular valve (AV). The morphologic right ventricle is trabeculated with the moderator band visible at its apex and an infundibulum (outlet component) that separates the tricuspid valve (with three leaflets and septal attachments) and the semilunar valve. Tricuspid annulus is closer to the apex than the mitral valve annulus. On the other hand, the morphologic left ventricle is smooth and there is direct continuity between the mitral valve (with two leaflets and without septal attachment) and the semilunar valve because of the absence of an infundibulum. In a right ventricular loop (D loop), the morphologic right ventricular sinus (inflow) lies to the right of the morphologic left ventricle whereas in a left ventricular loop (L loop) the morphologic right ventricular sinus (inflow) lies to the left of the morphologic left ventricle (Fig. 2.**4**).

Identification and position of the great arteries will be determined on transverse images. The aorta gives rise to brachiocephalic arteries and coronary arteries whereas pulmonary artery bifurcates in right and left pulmonary branches. In the normal situation the aorta is posterior and to the right of the pulmonary artery. In D transposition or malposition, the aorta is anterior and to the right of the pulmonary artery and in L transposition or malposition, the aorta is anterior and to the left of the pulmonary artery (Fig. 2.**5**).

Then, atrioventricular and ventriculoarterial connections will be identified with the notions of concordance and discordance at each level. This will be achieved by using the different imaging planes. For example, atrioventricular connection is concordant

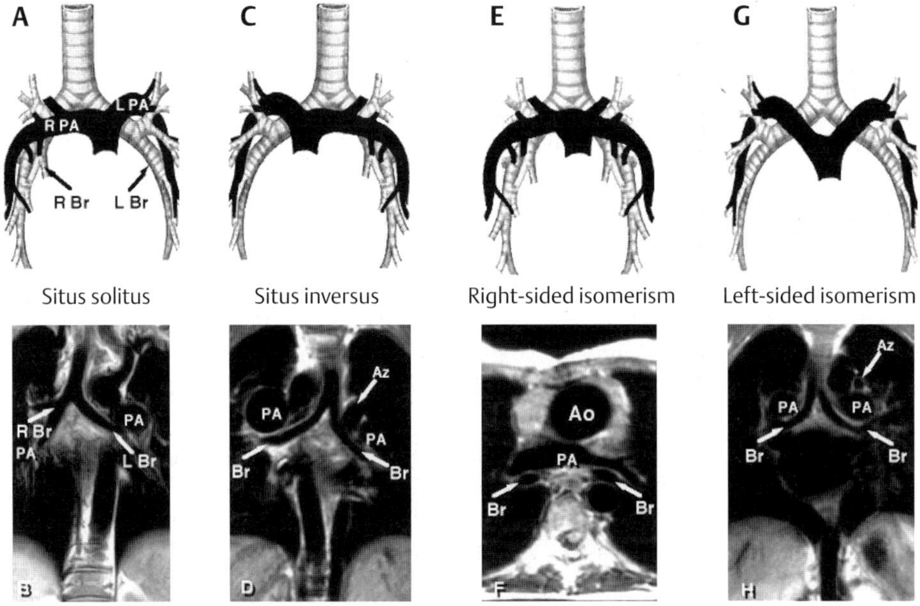

Fig. 2.**3** Schema and coronal and transverse spin-echo images demonstrate the different types of atrial situs in displaying morphology and relationship of the main bronchi and pulmonary arteries. The morphologically right main bronchus (R Br) is short and vertical, whereas the morphologically left main bronchus (L Br) is longer and more horizontal. The right pulmonary artery (RPA) courses anterior then lateral to the right bronchus whereas the left pulmonary artery (LPA) courses over the left bronchus. Atrial situs solitus is defined in **A** and **B**. In **C** and **D**, the morphologically left bronchus and left pulmonary artery are right-sided, and this indicates atrial situs inversus. In **E**, **F**, **G** and **H**, the bronchi and the pulmonary arteries show similar morphology. This indicates atrial situs ambiguous. Bilateral right main bronchi and right pulmonary arteries indicate right-sided isomerism (in **E** and **F** in a patient with pulmonary atresia) whereas bilateral left main bronchi and left pulmonary arteries suggest left-sided isomerism (**G**, **H**). Azygos vein continuation (Az) is more often encountered in left-sided isomerism (**H**) but can exist with situs inversus (**D**).

when the morphologically right atrium is connected to the morphologically right ventricle.

For ventriculoarterial connections, depending on anatomic features while considering or not considering the infundibulum and the conus arteriosus as a similar structure, there are four possible situations (Fig. 2.**6**).

1. Concordant ventriculoarterial connections when a morphologically right ventricle is connected to the pulmonary artery with an isolated subpulmonary conus responsible for discontinuity between tricuspid valve and pulmonary artery and a morphologically left ventricle is connected to the aorta with mitro-aortic continuity. These are the normal connections.
2. Discordant ventriculoarterial connections when a morphologically right ventricle is connected to the aorta with an isolated subaortic conus responsible for disconti-

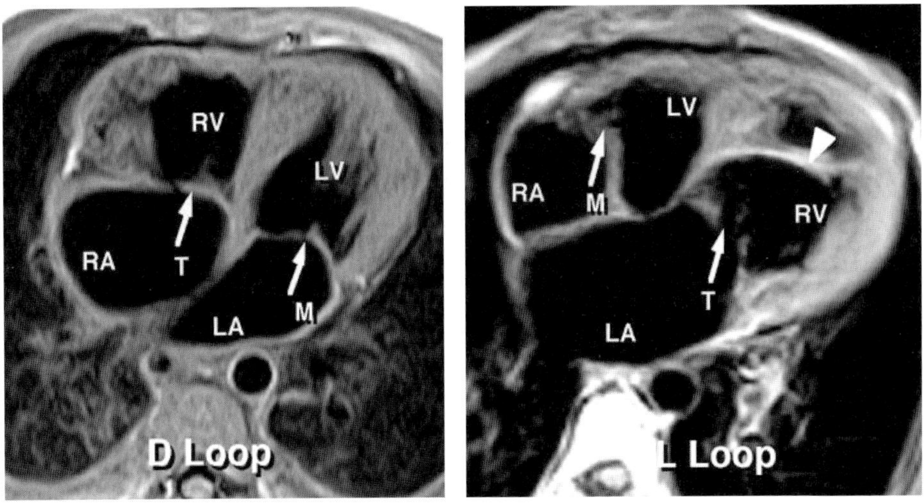

Fig. 2.4 Transverse spin-echo images (four cavities view) allow determination of the ventricular loop. Each ventricle will be identified by its own morphology and by its atrioventricular valve (AV). The morphologic right ventricle (RV) is trabeculated with the moderator band visible at its apex (arrow-head). Tricuspid annulus (T) is closer to the apex than the mitral valve annulus (M). On the other hand, the morphologic left ventricle is smooth. In a right ventricular loop (D loop), the morphologic right ventricular sinus (inflow) lies to the right of the morphologic left ventricle whereas in a left ventricular loop (L loop) the morphologic right ventricular sinus (inflow) lies to the left of the morphologic left ventricle.

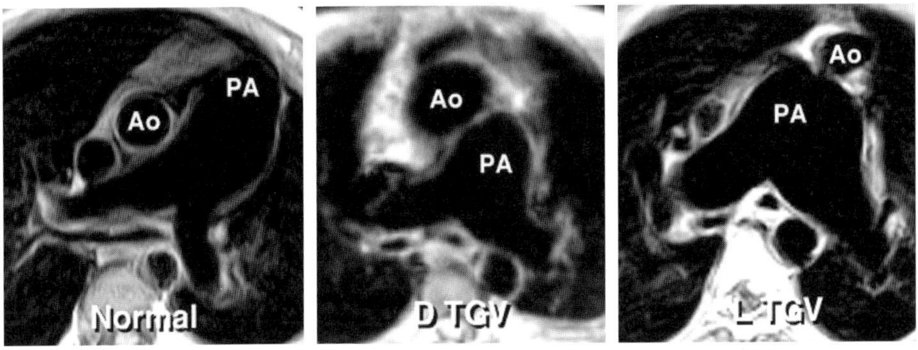

Fig. 2.5 Identification and position of the great arteries are determined on transverse images. The aorta (Ao) gives rise to brachiocephalic arteries and coronary arteries whereas the pulmonary artery (PA) bifurcates in right and left pulmonary branches. In the normal situation the aorta is posterior and to the right of the pulmonary artery. In D transposition or malposition, the aorta is anterior and to the right of the pulmonary artery and in L transposition or malposition, the aorta is anterior and to the left of the pulmonary artery.

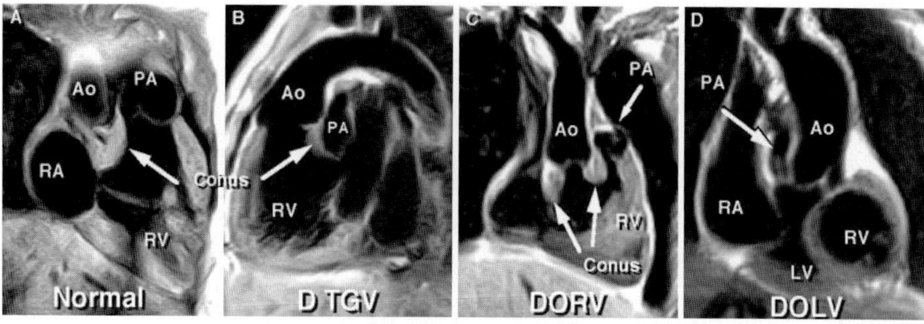

Fig. 2.**6** Ventriculoarterial connections and different types of conus. **A** represents the normal connections with a morphologically right ventricle (RV) connected to the pulmonary artery (PA) with an isolated subpulmonary conus responsible for discontinuity between tricuspid valve and pulmonary artery. **B** represents a discordant ventriculoarterial connection with a morphologically RV connected to the aorta (Ao) with an isolated subaortic conus responsible for discontinuity between tricuspid valve and aorta. This is the situation encountered in D transposition of the great vessels (D TGV). **C** and **D** represent double ventriculoarterial connections with both great vessels arising from the same ventricle. This is the case of double outlet right ventricle (DORV) with a bilateral conus and double discontinuity (**C**) and double outlet left ventricle (DOLV) with absence of conus (**D**).

nuity between tricuspid valve and aorta and a morphologically left ventricle is connected to the pulmonary artery with continuity between the mitral valve and pulmonary artery. This is the situation encountered in D transposition of the great vessels.

3. Double ventriculoarterial connections when both great vessels arise from the same ventricle. This is the case of a double outlet right ventricle with a bilateral conus and double discontinuity and double outlet left ventricle, a rare situation with absence of conus.
4. Single ventriculoarterial connection when there is a common arterial trunk and in cases of pulmonary or aortic atresia.

In complex cases, especially in malposed heart, one can follow the loop rule of R. Van Praagh: right ventricle and aorta are situated on the same side in 95% of normal and abnormal hearts (Fig. 2.**7**). A right ventricular loop is associated with the aorta situated on the right of the pulmonary artery and conversely [41].

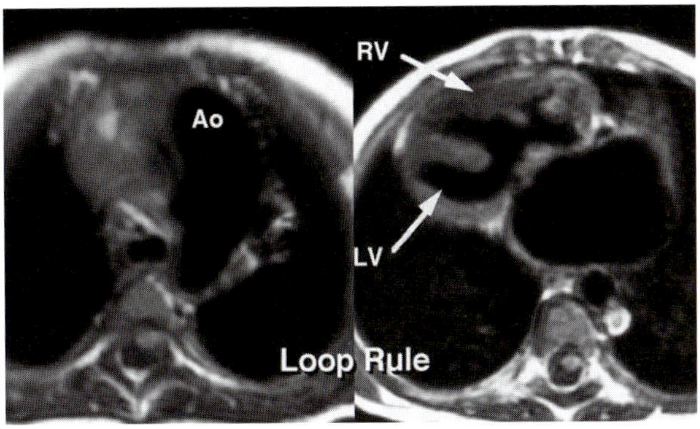

Fig. 2.7 Loop rule: the right ventricle (RV) and the aorta (Ao) are situated on the same side in 95% of normal and abnormal hearts. In this example of complex malformation with dextrocardia, there is a left ventricular loop: the morphologic RV lies to the left of the morphologic left ventricle (LV). It is associated with the aorta situated anterior and on the left of the pulmonary artery (L malposition).

2.4 Thoracic Aortic and Aortic Arch Anomalies

Congenital anomalies of the aorta and aortic arch are described in the Chapter 3 of this book and illustrated in the second section of the companion CD-ROM.

2.5 Cono-Truncal Malformations and Complex Anomalies

Echocardiography and angiography may be limited in the preoperative evaluation of cono-truncal malformations and complex diseases. Numerous studies have demonstrated the contribution of MRI in the description of these anomalies [42–47]. In these complex anomalies it is essential to image the heart with three tomographic planes: transverse, coronal and oblique sagittal. The goal of different MR imaging techniques in these anomalies will be to demonstrate the following features:

1. The segmental description and connections in complex anomalies, particularly the relationship of the great vessels.
2. Presence, site and degree of pulmonary stenosis.
3. Presence, size, stenosis and connections of pulmonary artery branches.
4. Assessment of ventricular chambers size, position and size of the VSD, atrioventricular valves.
5. Evaluation of associated systemic collaterals.
6. Presence or absence of pulmonary trunk and pulmonary confluence in pulmonary atresia.
7. Palliative shunt patency.
8. Post-operative complications after surgery.
9. Connections of pulmonary and systemic veins and associated anomalous venous vessel course in the thorax.

Cono-truncal malformations comprise the tetralogy of Fallot, pulmonary atresia, double outlet right and left ventricles, truncus arteriosus and transposition of the great arteries.

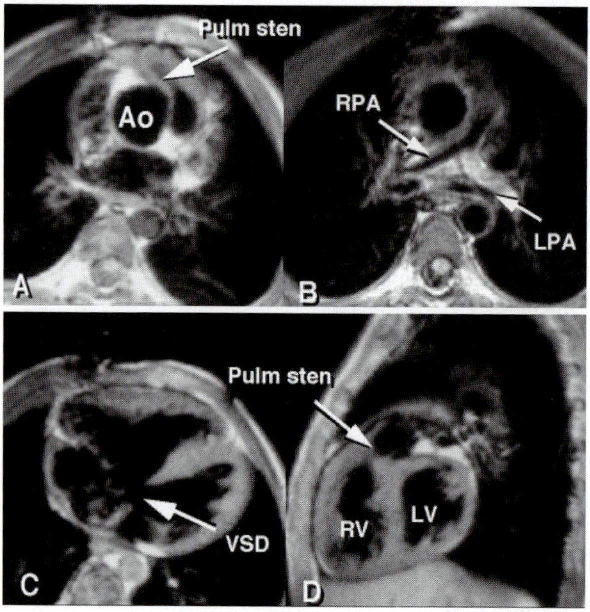

Fig. 2.**8** Tetralogy of Fallot. Transverse (**A**, **B**, **C**) and sagittal (**D**) images demonstrate an enlarged aorta (Ao) just above a large ventricular septal defect (VSD). The pulmonary stenosis (pulm sten) is mainly infundibular. It is associated with a severe hypoplasia of the pulmonary trunk and right (RPA) and left (LPA) pulmonary branches and right ventricular (RV) hypertrophy.

2.5.1 Tetralogy of Fallot

The tetralogy of Fallot, including right ventricular outflow obstruction, malalignment ventricular septal defect (VSD), overriding aorta and right ventricular hypertrophy is due to underdevelopment of the infundibulum (subpulmonary conus) with anterior, superior and leftward displacement of the parietal band (crista supraventricularis). This displacement is responsible for narrowing of the right ventricular outflow tract and leads to underdevelopment of the pulmonary valve, pulmonary trunk and pulmonary arteries and for overriding the VSD by the aortic root [44,48]. Associated anomalies are: right aortic arch (25%), abnormal origin and course of coronary arteries and muscular VSDs.

The site and degree of pulmonary obstruction and hypoplasia can be demonstrated on transverse and sagittal images. The size of the main pulmonary artery and pulmonary branches is the most important information provided by transverse and coronal MR images. In cases of severe narrowing of the right ventricular outflow tract and pulmonary arteries, transverse and coronal planes are essential to recognize the presence and size of systemic collaterals. The degree of aortic overriding (displaced anteriorly and rightward), the size of the VSD and the right ventricular enlargement and hypertrophy will also be determined from the three orthogonal tomograms (Fig. 2.**8**).

2.5.2 Pulmonary Atresia

Pulmonary atresia is defined as an interruption of the continuity between the right ventricular chamber and the main pulmonary artery. The infundibular portion of the right ventricle ends blindly and is usually hypoplastic. The main pulmonary artery is

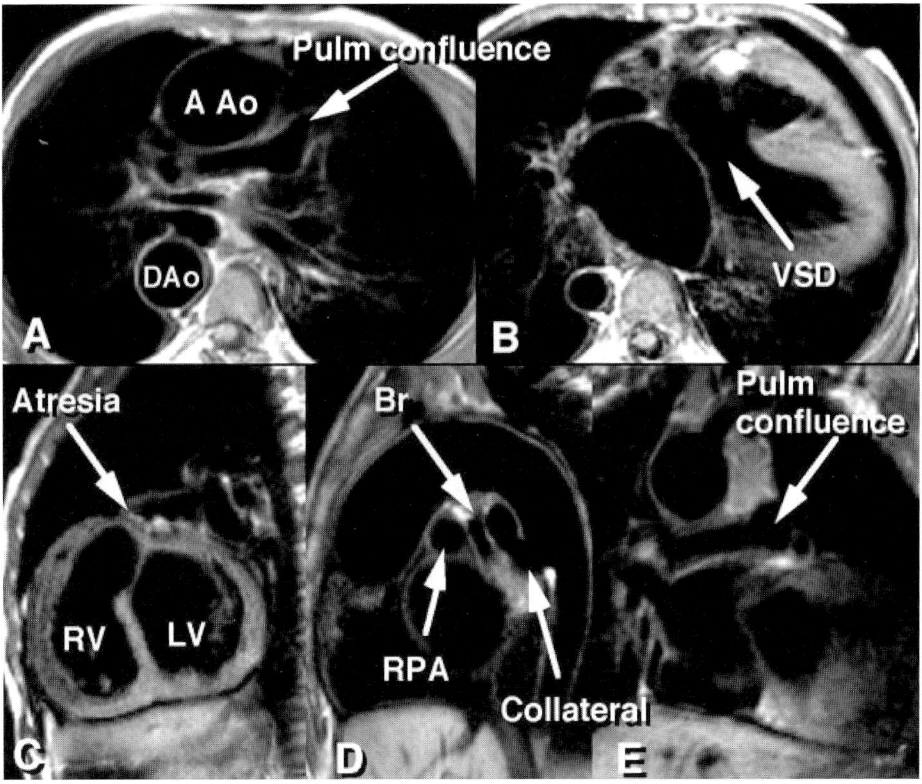

Fig. 2.**9** Transverse (**A**, **B**), sagittal oblique (**C**, **D**) and coronal (**E**) spin-echo images in a patient with pulmonary atresia. The atresia appears as medium signal intensity tissue separating the right ventricular outflow tract (RV) and the pulmonary artery on the sagittal image (**C**). Pulmonary trunk and central pulmonary confluence are demonstrated as well (**A**, **E**). Sagittal image (**D**) shows a large systemic collateral arising from the descending aorta, situated behind the bronchus (Br) whereas the right pulmonary artery (RPA) is situated in front. There is a large aortic root (A Ao) overriding a large malalignment ventricular septal defect (VSD) and there is a right aortic arch.

underdeveloped or atretic and right and left pulmonary arteries are often also hypoplastic. The most important element in pulmonary atresia is to demonstrate the presence of central confluence of the pulmonary arteries even when the main pulmonary artery is absent in order to determine the feasibility of surgical repair. MRI is the best method to show this confluence because of its multiplanar capability [49]. Diagnosis of pulmonary atresia relies upon the demonstration of a high and/or medium signal intensity tissue separating the right ventricular outflow tract and the pulmonary artery, particularly on transverse and sagittal images. Usually a large malalignment VSD is also present and well demonstrated in several planes (Fig. 2.**9**). Collateral blood supply to the lungs is made by enlarged bronchial and intercostal arteries or a patent ductus arteriosus. Demonstration of these systemic collaterals is crucial for surgery in order to include ligation of these vessels during the procedure. These vessels can be differentiated from pulmonary arteries on transverse and coronal images because

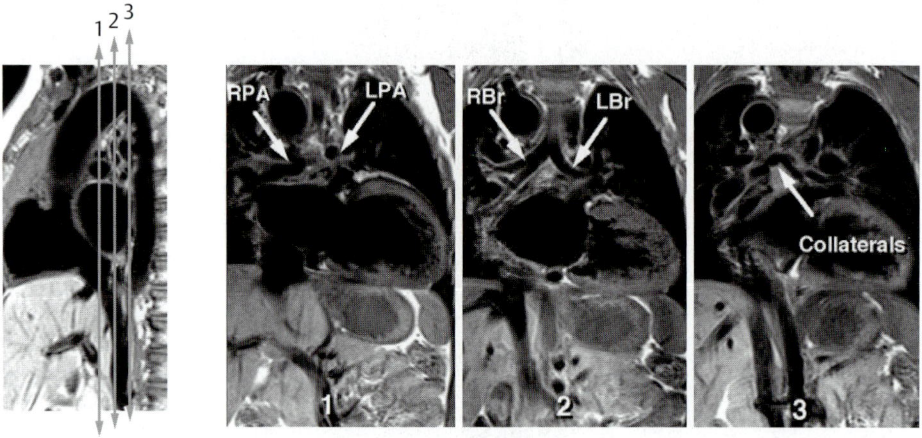

Fig. 2.**10** Demonstration of the systemic collaterals in a patient with pulmonary atresia. The collaterals can be differentiated from the right and left pulmonary arteries (RPA, LPA) on transverse and coronal images because they usually are located posterior to the right and left main bronchi (RBr, LBr) whereas the pulmonary arteries are located anteriorly.

they usually are located posterior to the main bronchi whereas pulmonary arteries are located anteriorly [45] (Fig. 2.**10**).

2.5.3 Double Outlet Right Ventricle

Double outlet right ventricle (DORV) is defined as follows: both the aorta and the pulmonary artery arise completely or nearly completely from the morphologic right ventricle. The only way of left ventricular ejection relies on the presence of a VSD. Clinical presentation depends upon the presence of pulmonary stenosis. If it is present, cyanosis occurs as in the tetralogy of Fallot, if not, presentation is similar to a large left-to-right shunt. Two features are important in DORV: the position of the great vessels and the position and size of the associated malalignment VSD and their relationship (commitment) in order to plan the surgical approach. Classically, the great vessels have a side-by-side relationship and there is a bilateral conus (subaortic and subpulmonary) well demonstrated on coronal images. But various degrees of malposition may be present. The bilateral conus is responsible for discontinuity between the atrioventricular and semilunar valves. This double discontinuity, when it is present, allows one to differentiate DORV from D transposition of the great vessels (continuity between mitral and pulmonary valve) and tetralogy of Fallot (continuity between mitral and aortic valve). The VSD can be subaortic (aortic commitment) allowing internal repair by intraventricular baffle when pulmonary stenosis is not severe, subpulmonary (Taussig-Bing anomaly) which requires a markedly different surgical approach or doubly committed (subaortic and subpulmonary) [41]. MRI is a unique tool to image the exact location of the great vessels and the commitment of

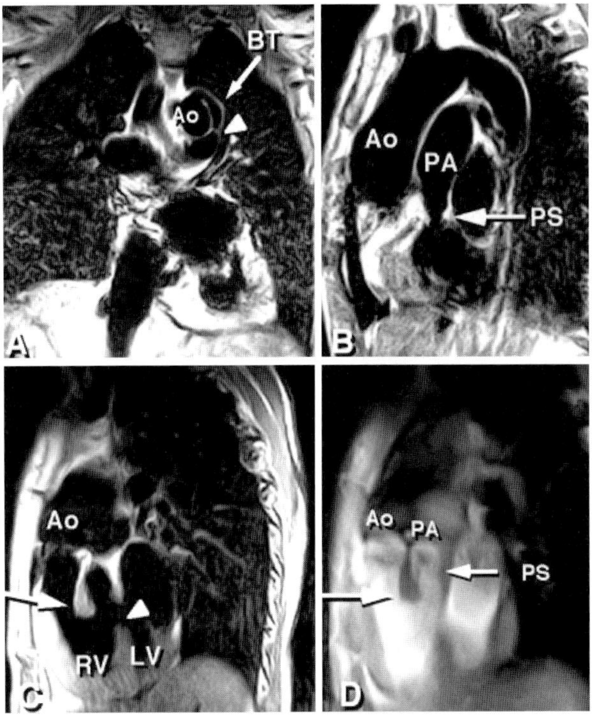

Fig. 2.**11** Spin-echo (**A**, **B**, **C**) and cine-GE (**D**) images of a patient with double outlet right ventricle and pulmonary stenosis. A Blalock-Taussig shunt (BT) has been realized on the left pulmonary artery (**A**). A stenosis is visualized at the anastomosis (arrow-head on **A**). Aorta (Ao) is anterior to the pulmonary artery (PA) but both great vessels arise from the right ventricle (RV). There is a double conus, subaortic and subpulmonary (arrow on **C** and **D**) and a large ventricular septal defect (arrow-head on **C**). A valvular pulmonary stenosis (PS) is well demonstrated on the sagittal images.

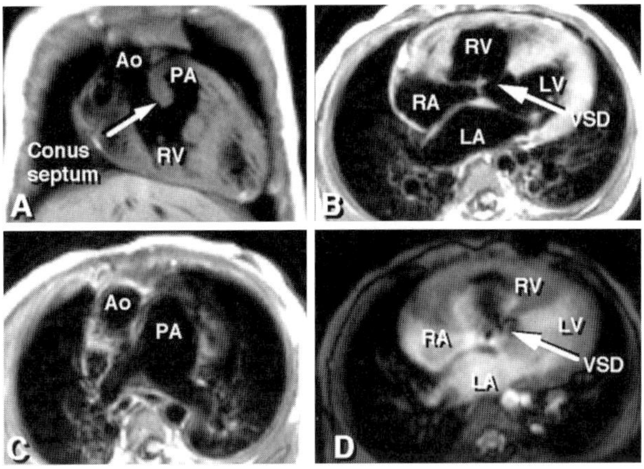

Fig. 2.**12** Coronal (**A**) and transverse (**B**, **C**, **D**) spin-echo and cine-GE images of a patient with double outlet right ventricle and subpulmonary ventricular septal defect (VSD) (Taussig-Bing anomaly). The great vessels (Ao, PA) are positioned side by side (D malposition) on transverse image (**C**). The VSD is subpulmonary committed. An internal baffle connecting left ventricle to the aorta will be impossible. Coronal image shows the side-by-side relationship of the great vessels and the conus septum between the great arteries. Cine-GE image (**D**) shows the turbulent flow coming from the left ventricle (LV) across the VSD.

the VSD [1, 2, 42, 47] (Figs. 2.**11** and 2.**12**). In the rare situation where both great arteries arise from the morphologic left ventricle (double outlet left ventricle), usually associated with a left ventricular loop, there is absence of subaortic and subpulmonary conus (Fig. 2.**13**).

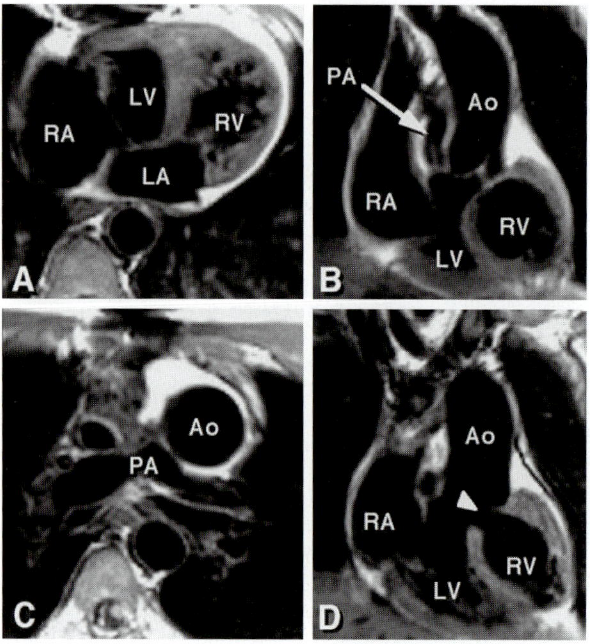

Fig. 2.**13** Spin-echo images of a patient with double outlet left ventricle, pulmonary stenosis and ventricular septal defect (VSD). The aorta (Ao) is anterior and to the left of the pulmonary artery (PA) (L malposition) on transverse image (**C**). Both great vessels arise from a morphologically left ventricle. There is a L loop and atrioventricular discordance. The right atrium (RA) is connected to a morphologically left ventricle (LV) whereas the left atrium (LA) is connected to a morphologically right ventricle (RV). The VSD is subaortic (arrowhead). There is no conus between the great arteries and the LV.

2.5.4 Truncus Arteriosus

Truncus arteriosus is defined as a single arterial trunk arising from the heart and distributing the blood flow to the coronary arteries, the pulmonary arteries and the aorta. The truncus overrides both ventricles and a large malaligned VSD and the truncal valve is often malformed. The classification of the different types of truncus arteriosus relies upon the branching pattern into the pulmonary and aortic circulation pathways [50]. Type I is the most frequent where there is a common main pulmonary artery arising from the lateral or posterior border of the truncus and dividing rapidly into right and left pulmonary arteries well demonstrated on transverse, sagittal and coronal images (Fig. 2.**14**). Type II is characterized by both the right and left pulmonary arteries arising separately from the truncus. In type III only one of the pulmonary branches (usually the right) originates from the truncus, the other one arising from a persistent patent ductus arteriosus or a systemic collateral from the aorta (Fig. 2.**15**). Type IV is the association of a type I with aortic arch interruption where the descending aorta is perfused through a large patent ductus arteriosus (Fig. 2.**16**). The right aortic arch is frequently associated (25%). MRI is invaluable to demonstrate these different branching patterns with the help of the three different spin-echo planes described previously and a coronal cine image centered on truncal valve will assess the degree of valvular incompetence, frequently associated [47,49].

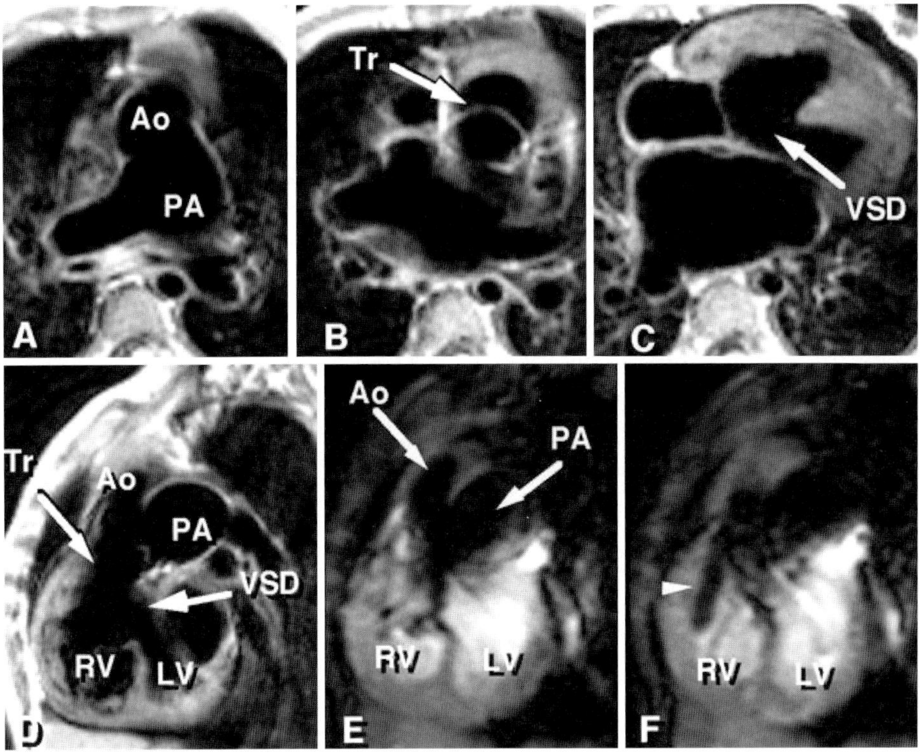

Fig. 2.**14** Transverse (**A**, **B**, **C**) and sagittal oblique (**D**, **E**, **F**) spin-echo images of a patient with a type I truncus arteriosus. The common main pulmonary artery (PA) arises from the truncus then bifurcates into right and left pulmonary arteries (**A**, **B**). A large ventricular septal defect (VSD) lies below the truncal vessel. Sagittal spin-echo (**D**) and cine-GE (**E**, **F**) images demonstrate the truncal bifurcation, the distribution of turbulent flow in both the PA and the aorta (Ao) in systole (**E**) and the regurgitation of the truncal valve in diastole (arrow-head on **F**).

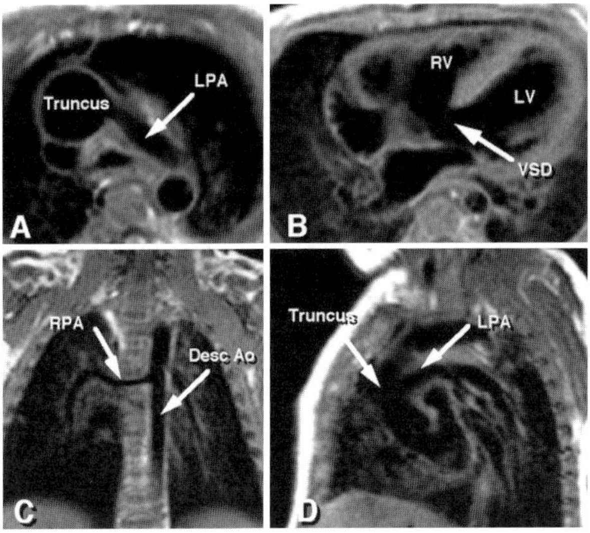

Fig. 2.**15** Type III truncus arteriosus. The left pulmonary artery (LPA) originates directly from the truncus whereas the right pulmonary artery (RPA) arises from a systemic collateral coming from the descending aorta (Desc Ao). A large malalignment ventricular septal defect (VSD) lies below the truncus.

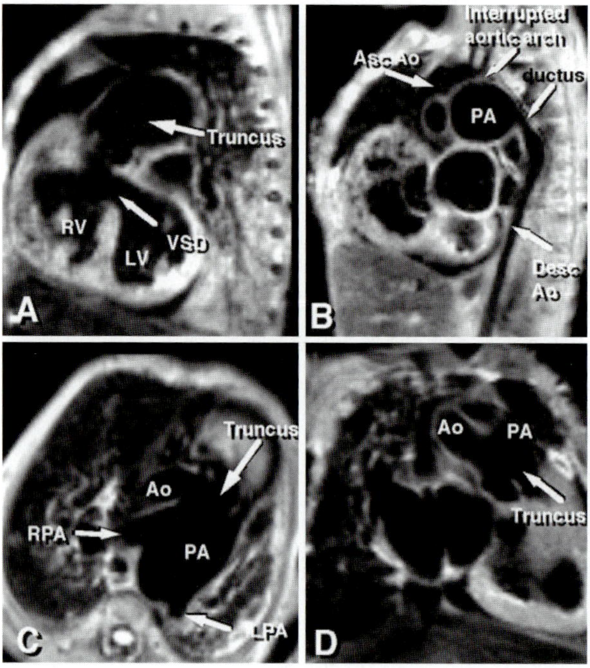

Fig. 2.**16** Type IV truncus arteriosus (type I with interruption of the aortic arch). The common main pulmonary artery (PA) arises from the truncus then bifurcates into right and left (RPA, LPA) pulmonary arteries (**C**, **D**). A large ventricular septal defect (VSD) lies below the truncal vessel overriding the defect (**A**). Sagittal image (**B**) demonstrates the hypoplastic ascending and horizontal aorta just above the interruption of the aortic arch and the connection between the pulmonary artery and the descending aorta through a large patent ductus arteriosus (ductus).

2.5.5 Transposition of the Great Arteries

Transposition of the great arteries (TGA) means that each great artery arises completely from the wrong ventricle: aorta arising from a morphologic right ventricle and pulmonary artery arising from a morphologic left ventricle. In D-TGA there is atrioventricular concordance and ventriculoarterial discordance. Transverse images demonstrate easily the aorta located anteriorly, originating from the normally positioned right ventricle and to the right of the pulmonary artery, originating from the posterior morphologic left ventricle and which is recognized by its bifurcation. The aortic valve is located superiorly due to the presence of a subaortic conus and is responsible for the tricuspid-aortic discontinuity while the absence of a subpulmonary conus realizes pulmonary-mitral continuity. In TGA, the right ventricle is the systemic ventricle and is responsible for posterior bulging of the ventricular septum on sagittal images (Fig. 2.**17**) [47].

In L-TGA the aorta is located anteriorly and to the left of the pulmonary artery. It could be isolated or a part of a congenitally corrected transposition where there is atrioventricular and ventriculoarterial discordance. In this case and without associated malformations a hemodynamically normal heart exists. The right atrium is connected to a morphologic left ventricle (L loop) then to the pulmonary artery and the left atrium is connected to a morphologic right ventricle then to the aorta (see Fig. 2.**13**).

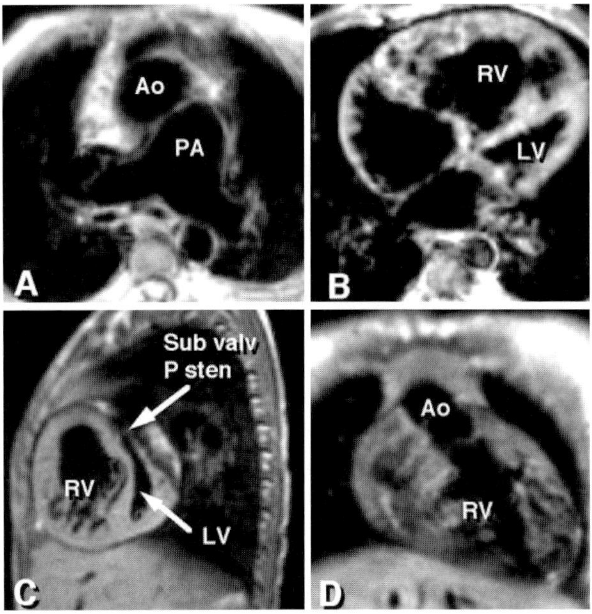

Fig. 2.**17** D-transposition of the great arteries with subvalvular pulmonary stenosis (Sub valv P sten). Transverse (**A**, **B**) and coronal (**D**) images demonstrate easily the aorta (Ao) located anteriorly originating from the normally positioned right ventricle (RV) and to the right of the pulmonary artery (PA), recognized by its bifurcation originating from the posterior morphologic left ventricle (LV). The subpulmonary obstruction is dynamic due to posterior bulging of the interventricular septum well demonstrated on sagittal image (**C**).

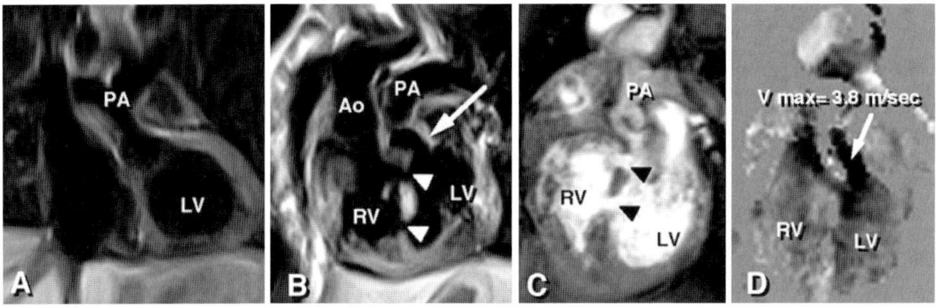

Fig. 2.**18** D-Transposition of the great arteries with pulmonary stenosis (arrow) and perimembranous and muscular ventricular septal defects (arrow-heads). Coronal image (**A**) demonstrates the abnormal connection of the left ventricle (LV) with the pulmonary artery (PA), recognized by its bifurcation. The sagittal spin-echo (**B**), cine-GE (**C**) and velocity-encoded (**D**) images show the valvular and subvalvular pulmonary stenosis due to a fibromuscular tunnel and the presence of a subaortic conus, responsible for tricuspid-aortic discontinuity. On **D**, the velocity was encoded superiorly and allowed the measurement of a maximum velocity of 3.8 m/sec corresponding to a pressure gradient of 58 mmHg by using the modified Bernoulli equation.

Associated anomalies with TGA are: VSD, pulmonary stenosis, patent ductus arteriosus and Ebstein's anomaly of the left-sided atrioventricular valve in corrected TGA.

VSD is usually a perimembranous VSD. It can be associated with a muscular VSD (Fig. 2.**18**). Pulmonary stenosis may be valvular and/or subvalvular (Fig. 2.**19**). The left ventricular outflow tract obstruction may be organic with the presence of a subpul-

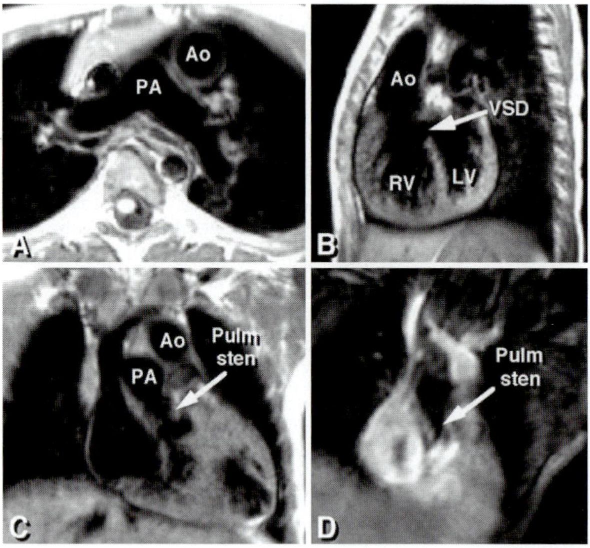

Fig. 2.**19** L-Transposition of the great arteries with pulmonary stenosis (Pulm sten) and perimembranous ventricular septal defect (VSD). Transverse (**A**) and sagittal (**B**) images show the aorta (Ao) located anteriorly originating from the normally positioned right ventricle (RV) and to the left of the pulmonary artery (PA), recognized by its bifurcation originating from the posterior morphologic left ventricle (LV). Coronal images (**C**, **D**) demonstrate the valvular and subvalvular pulmonary stenosis with the flow void originating from the subvalvular region on the cine-GE image (**D**).

monary membrane or a fibromuscular tunnel or dynamic due to posterior bulging of the interventricular septum, well demonstrated on sagittal spin-echo and cine images in systole (see Fig. 2.**17**).

2.5.6 Single Ventricle

Single ventricle anomaly (double inlet ventricle) is a complex anomaly where both atria connect to only one ventricular chamber by a single or two atrioventricular valves. Usually, a rudimentary chamber, which has no inlet component, communicates with the main chamber by a VSD called the bulboventricular foramen but it may be absent. Among the four types of single ventricles described by R. Van Praagh, type A (morphologically left main chamber) is the most frequent, type B (morphologically right main chamber) is less frequent and type C and type D (main ventricular chamber impossible to characterize as left or right) are rare [51]. Frequent associated findings are pulmonary atresia and malposition of the great vessels. In this type of complex anomalies, MRI is very helpful and the use of the three planes (transverse, coronal and sagittal) is usually necessary, particularly in demonstrating the type of the main chamber and associated anomalies for surgical planning [7,52]. The following three criteria will be used to define the morphological main chamber.

1. The pattern of the chamber: if it is smooth, it will suggest a left ventricular morphology of the main chamber, if it is trabeculated, it will suggest a right ventricular morphology of the main chamber.

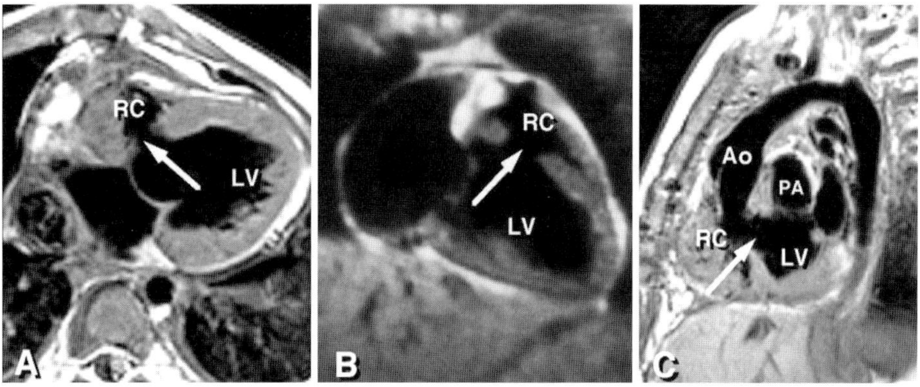

Fig. 2.**20** Type A single ventricle, L malposition of the great vessels and single atrioventricular valve. The main chamber is a left ventricular (LV) type chamber. The rudimentary chamber (RC) is located anterosuperiorly, communicates with the main chamber by the bulboventricular foramen (arrow) and is connected to the aorta (Ao), anterior and to the left of the pulmonary artery (PA).

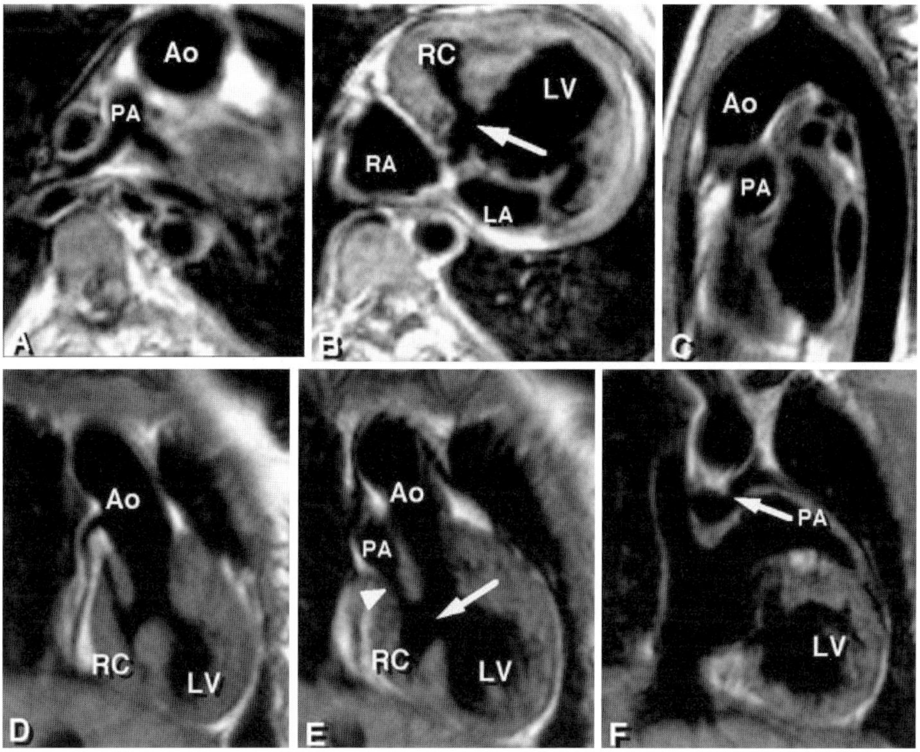

Fig. 2.**21** Type A single ventricle, L malposition of the great vessels (**A**) and severe subpulmonary stenosis (arrow-head). The main chamber is a left ventricular (LV) type chamber. The rudimentary chamber (RC) is located anterosuperiorly, communicates with the main chamber by the bulboventricular foramen (arrow) and is connected to both the aorta (Ao), and the pulmonary artery (PA). The pulmonary confluence is well visualized on transverse and coronal images (**A**, **F**) and the pulmonary branches are hypoplastic.

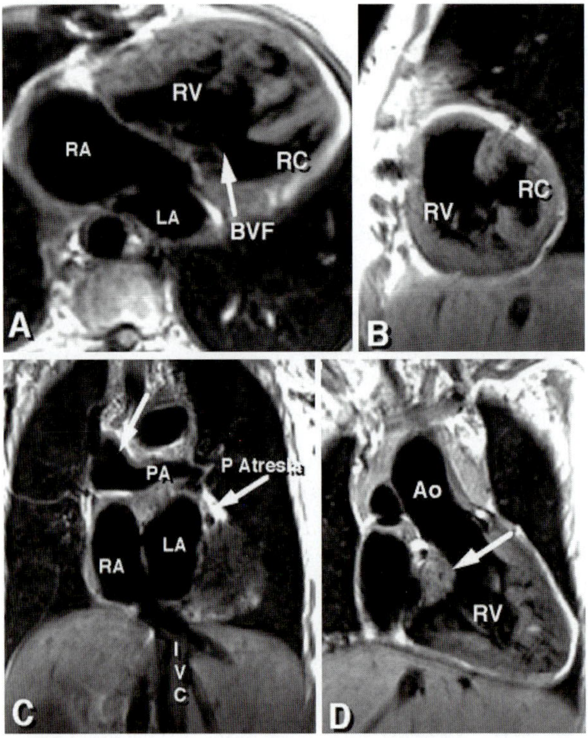

Fig. 2.**22** Type B single ventricle with situs ambiguus, complete AV canal and pulmonary atresia. The main chamber is a right ventricular (RV) type chamber with trabeculations and presence of an infundibulum (arrow on **D**) in the main chamber. The rudimentary chamber (RC) is located posterior and inferior and communicates with the main chamber by the bulboventricular foramen (BVF). The pulmonary confluence (PA) is well demonstrated on coronal image (**C**) and the pulmonary atresia appears as high signal intensity between the dominant chamber and the pulmonary confluence. The patient underwent a cavopulmonary shunt (arrow on **C**).

2. The position of the rudimentary chamber: if it is located anterior and superior, the main chamber is of left type (Figs. 2.**20** and 2.**21**) whereas if it is located posterior and inferior, the main chamber is of right type (Fig. 2.**22**).
3. The presence or absence of an infundibulum in the main chamber: the presence of an infundibulum separating the atrioventricular valves and the adjacent semilunar valve will be suggestive of a morphologically right main chamber and conversely.

2.5.7 Tricuspid Atresia

Tricuspid atresia is a rare cyanotic malformation where the right atrioventricular valve is not patent and is replaced by muscular, fibrous or fat tissue in the atrioventricular groove and there is no direct communication between the right atrium and the right ventricle, which is hypoplastic. In all cases there is an interatrial communication (patent foramen ovale or a true ostium secundum atrial septal defect) and often a VSD. The great vessels may be in the normal position or transposed. The pulmonary tract may be normal, stenosed or hypoplastic. The obstruction can be subpulmonary due to a restrictive VSD. The most frequent form is tricuspid atresia with normally positioned great vessels, pulmonary stenosis and small VSD [53]. Diagnosis is made on a transverse spin-echo image where the atretic valve is characterized by an area of medium to high signal intensity in the right atrioventricular groove and the absence of flow between the enlarged right atrium and the hypoplastic right ventricle on the corresponding cine image (see Fig. 2.**39**). The associated atrial septal defect and VSD will also be demonstrated on transverse images.

2.6 Pulmonary and Systemic Venous Anomalies

MRI is particularly suitable for the evaluation of pulmonary and systemic venous anomalies because of the large field of view and multi-oblique imaging capability [2, 9]. Demonstration of a left superior vena cava (L SVC) as well as azygos continuation is easy and of importance in surgical planning, particularly in cases of functional single ventricle (single ventricle, tricuspid atresia) where cavopulmonary shunts can be considered. The L SVC draining the left subclavian vein and the left internal jugular vein descends vertically in front of the aortic arch, then penetrates the pericardium and approaches the posterior atrioventricular sulcus, receives the great cardiac vein and becomes the coronary sinus connecting to the right atrium (Fig. 2.**23A**). Persistent L SVC can be a part of bilateral superior vena caval system. The left innominate vein can be present (bridging innominate) or absent. Rarely, the right superior vena cava may be absent. L SVC is often associated with tetralogy of Fallot, ventricular septal defects, sinus venosus atrial septal defect, cyanotic cardiac malformations and complex anomalies with viscero-atrial situs ambiguous.

When the suprarenal inferior vena cava (IVC) is absent, venous drainage of the lower body is done via a dilated azygos or hemiazygos vein (Fig. 2.**23B**). Azygos continuation frequently associated with left atrial isomerism and polysplenia appears as a venous structure running in the paravertebral space, then running up in the thorax either on the left or the right side. It is associated with a separate entry of the hepatic veins into the right atrium.

The rare anomalous drainage of the IVC in the left atrium will be demonstrated on transverse and sagittal images (Fig. 2.**23D**).

Other rare systemic venous anomalies (such as innominate vein coursing posterior to the aorta, which can be mistaken for the right pulmonary artery) will be only detected by MRI (Fig. **2.23C**).

Evaluation of the pulmonary venous connection is one of the weaknesses of both echocardiography and angiography whereas MRI plays an important role in identifying partial and total anomalous pulmonary venous connections, cor triatriatum and pulmonary vein stenosis [54]. The spin-echo imaging technique in multiple planes may demonstrate the anomaly but images can be suboptimal in cases of signal dropout due to a thin wall of the vein surrounded by the signal void of the lung. Gadolinium-enhanced breath-hold 3D MRA is at present the technique of choice to demonstrate these anomalies. With the help of two series, one early and one late, one can subtract the early series from the late one in order to keep the veins injected only. This

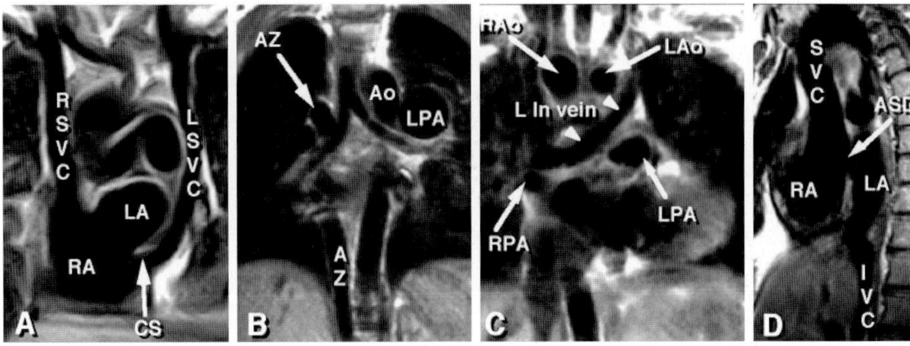

Fig. 2.**23** Systemic venous anomalies. **A**: Left superior vena cava (L SVC) is easily recognized as a vessel draining the left subclavian and the left internal jugular veins, descending vertically in front of the aortic arch, and becoming the coronary sinus (CS) connecting to the right atrium (RA). **B**: Azygos continuation (AZ) appears as a venous structure running in the paravertebral space, then running up in the thorax either on the left or the right side and joining the superior vena cava. **C**: Innominate vein (L In vein) coursing posterior to the aorta, which can be mistaken for the right pulmonary artery. **D**: Anomalous drainage of the inferior vena cava (IVC) in the left atrium is demonstrated on a sagittal image. It is associated with an atrial septal defect (ASD).

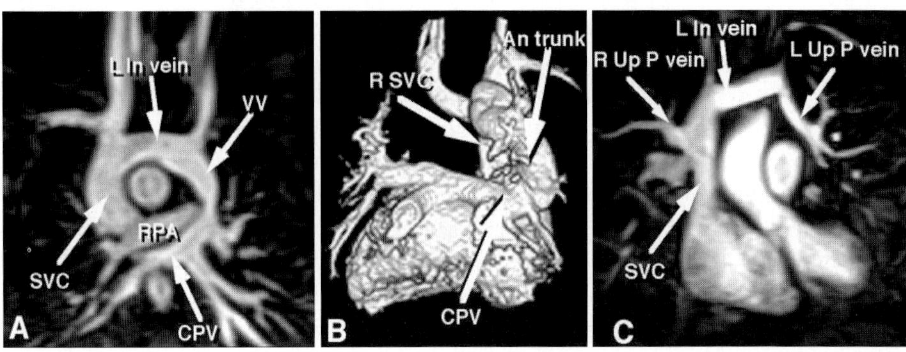

Fig. 2.**24** Pulmonary venous anomalies. **A**: Multiplanar reconstruction of MR angiography in a total anomalous pulmonary venous connection (TAPVC). The pulmonary veins join to form a confluence (CPV) posterior to the left atrium, then an anomalous vertical vein (VV) originating from this confluence joins the left innominate vein (L In Vein) then the superior vena cava (SVC). **B**: Posterior view of a surface rendering of MR angiography in a TAPVC. The pulmonary veins join to form a confluence (CPV) posterior to the left atrium, then an anomalous trunk (An trunk) originating from this confluence enters the posterior wall of right superior vena cava (R SVC). **C**: Multiplanar reconstruction of MR angiography in a partial anomalous pulmonary venous connection (PAPVC). The right upper pulmonary vein (R Up P vein) is connected to the superior vena cava (SVC) and the left upper pulmonary vein is connected to the left innominate vein (L In vein).

helps to differentiate the pulmonary veins from the arteries on the source images and reconstructions of MR angiography.

In total anomalous pulmonary venous connections (TAPVC), the pulmonary veins have no connections with the left atrium. All pulmonary veins from both lungs connect anomalously to the right atrium or to a systemic venous tributary. TAPVC is associated with major cardiac malformation in one-third of the cases.

There are four types of TAPVC.

1. Connection to the right atrium (15%): a common pulmonary vein draining both lungs or pulmonary veins draining separately into the postero-inferior portion of the right atrium.
2. Connection to the right common cardinal system (11%): the pulmonary veins join to form a confluence posterior to the left atrium, then an anomalous trunk originating from this confluence enters the posterior wall of right SVC (Fig. 2.**24B**).
3. Connection to the left common cardinal system:
   - Left innominate vein (36%): the pulmonary veins join to form a confluence posterior to the left atrium, then an anomalous trunk originating from this confluence (anomalous vertical vein) joins the left innominate vein then the SVC (Fig. 2.**24A**).
   - Coronary sinus (16%): The pulmonary veins join a common trunk, which connects to the coronary sinus in the region of the atrioventricular groove.
4. Connection to the umbilicovitelline system (13%): the pulmonary veins join to form a confluence behind the left atrium. Then, an anomalous trunk originating from this confluence penetrates the diaphragm and joins most commonly the portal vein at the confluence of the splenic and the superior mesenteric veins and less often the ductus venosus, one hepatic vein or the IVC.

In partial anomalous pulmonary venous connections (PAPVC), left-sided pulmonary veins usually connect to derivatives of the left cardinal system: coronary sinus and left innominate vein whereas right-sided pulmonary veins connect to derivatives of the right cardinal system: superior and inferior vena cava and right atrium.

The most frequent anomalous connections are: right pulmonary veins to superior vena cava, right pulmonary veins to right atrium or to the inferior vena cava (scimitar syndrome) and left pulmonary veins to left innominate vein (Fig. 2.**24C**). Right pulmonary veins with anomalous drainage to the superior vena cava is often associated with a sinus venosus atrial septal defect (see Fig. 2.**25A**). The veins from the whole lung or only the veins from the upper or lower lobes may be connected anomalously.

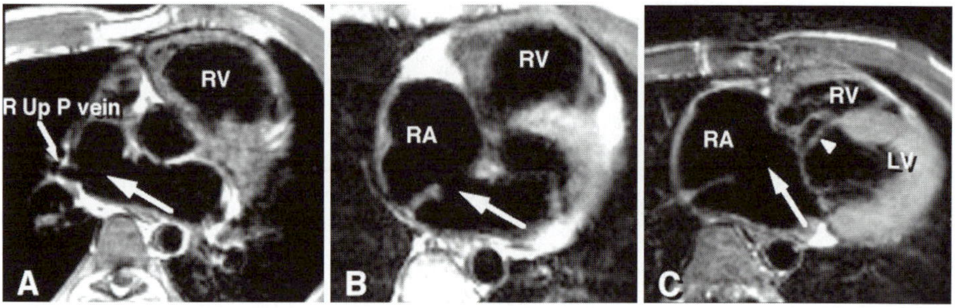

Fig. 2.**25** Different types of atrial septal defects (ASD). **A**: Sinus venosus ASD. The defect is located in the superior portion of the atrial septum at its junction with the superior vena cava (arrow) and very often associated with partial anomalous pulmonary vein drainage of the right upper pulmonary vein (R Up P vein). **B**: Ostium secundum ASD is the most frequent ASD found in the midportion of the atrial septum at the level of the fossa ovalis (arrow). **C**: Ostium primum ASD is a defect situated in the lower portion of the atrial septum, adjacent to the atrioventricular (AV) valves (arrow). It is often associated with abnormal chordal attachments of the AV valve to the crest of the ventricular septum (arrow-head).

2.7 Detection and Quantitative Analysis of Shunts, Stenoses and Regurgitations

One of the weaknesses of early MRI techniques was the difficulty to demonstrate thin anatomic structures such as the fossa ovalis and membranous septum because of signal dropout [55] (see Fig. 2.**1**). These are the sites where the defects are the most frequent. With recent advances in imaging techniques, the use of a large matrix (256 × 512) in multiple planes and cine-GE techniques allow better visualization of these regions and detection of flow voids due to left-to-right shunts [26]. However, several studies have demonstrated the efficiency of MRI in imaging the different portions of the atrial and ventricular septae with a sensitivity of 97 % and a specificity of 90 % in the detection of atrial septal defects (ASD) [56, 57]. Furthermore, VEC-MRI allows non-invasive quantification of pulmonary-to-systemic flow ratio (Qp/Qs) with a good correlation with echocardiographic and catheterization data and several studies have confirmed the accuracy of VEC-MRI for this purpose [34, 35]. However, two-dimensional and Doppler echocardiography are able to image the defects and quantify the shunts in numerous cases and MRI will be complementary to echocardiography when the findings are equivocal as well as in difficult cases and to confirm the importance of the shunt, thus avoiding the necessity for cardiac catheterization. This is the case in sinus venosus ASD where the defect is located in the superior portion of the atrial septum at its junction with the superior vena cava and very often associated with a partial anomalous pulmonary vein drainage (Fig. 2.**25 A**). Ostium secundum ASD is the most frequent ASD found in the midportion of the atrial septum at the level of the fossa ovalis. To assert the presence of the defect, it will be present in several adjacent images and in other imaging planes, usually the sagittal. As in echocardio-

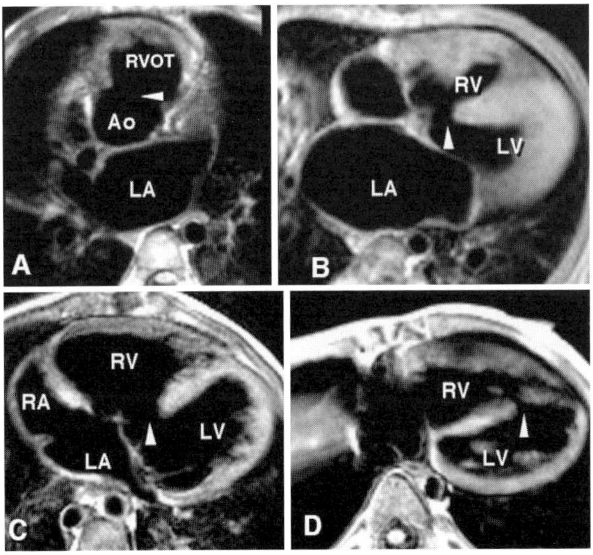

Fig. 2.26 Different types of ventricular septal defects (VSD). **A**: Infundibular or outlet VSD is situated immediately below the pulmonary valve (arrow-head). On transverse image it appears to directly connect the right ventricular outflow tract (RVOT) to the aorta (Ao). **B**: Large perimembranous VSD. The defect is situated just below the aortic root and extends to the superior portion of the inlet septum (arrow-head). **C**: Inlet VSD. The defect is adjacent to the atrioventricular (AV) valves (arrow-head) and is a component of a complete AV canal. Note the associated ostium primum ASD. **D**: Muscular VSD. The defect involves the muscular trabeculated septum (arrow-head).

graphy, one must find the increased thickness of the residual septum at the edges of the defect (Fig. 2.**25B**). Furthermore, cine-MR images centered at the same level confirm the presence of the defect in showing the flow void coming from the defect and extending into the right atrium due to a left-to-right shunt. Ostium primum ASD is a defect situated in the lower portion of the atrial septum, adjacent to the atrioventricular (AV) valves. This incomplete form of endocardial cushion defect is often associated with abnormal chordal attachments of the AV valve to the crest of the ventricular septum (Fig. 2.**25C**).

MRI was demonstrated to be particularly useful in the assessment of the interventricular septum and the different types of ventricular septal defects (VSD) (Fig. 2.**26**). Usually, the role of MRI in VSD is complementary to that of echocardiography in difficult cases [58,59,60]. One situation where MRI can bring additional information is in cases of outlet ventricular septal defect (VSD), where the defect is located immediately below the pulmonary valve and is often associated with an aortic regurgitation due to a prolapse of one of the sigmoid valves into the VSD. Demonstration of an intact membranous septum on coronal images as well as a vertical jet visualized on sagittal oblique cine-GE images allows the correct diagnosis (Fig. 2.**27**) and VEC-MRI allows the quantification of the shunt and the degree of associated aortic regurgitation. In this case, even if the shunt is moderate, surgery is necessary.

Patent ductus arteriosus remains difficult to image entirely in certain situations where the ductus is short or tortuous, even in a sagittal oblique plane encompassing aortic arch and pulmonary bifurcation (Fig. 2.**28**). MR angiography can help and estimation of pulmonary flow and the importance of a left-to-right shunt can be assessed

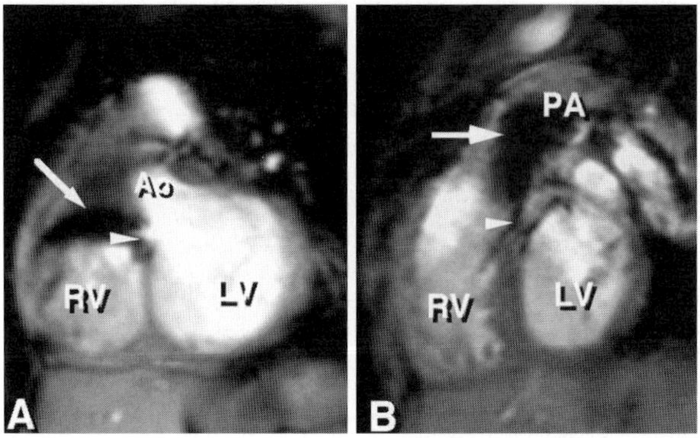

Fig. 2.**27** Sagittal oblique cine-GE images in a perimembranous (**A**) and an outlet (**B**) ventricular septal defect (VSD). In perimembranous VSD, the defect is located immediately below the aortic valve (arrowhead) and the flow void (left-to-right shunt) is horizontal (arrow). In outlet VSD, the defect is located immediately below the pulmonary valve (arrowhead) and the flow void (left-to-right shunt) is vertical. Ao = aorta, PA = pulmonary artery, RV = right ventricle, LV = left ventricle.

by measuring flow separately in the right and left pulmonary branches with VEC-MRI [37].

In patients with left-to-right shunts one major hemodynamic aspect is the determination of pulmonary pressure and resistances. The surgical decision depends on this evaluation. Some findings that are suggestive of pulmonary hypertension include right ventricular enlargement and hypertrophy, straightened or reversed curvature of the interventricular septum, dilatation of the pulmonary arteries and decrease or absence of the flow void at the level of the defect on cine-MR images. Decrease of flow in pulmonary branches with intravascular signals on spin-echo images has been demonstrated in patients with Eisenmenger's syndrome and shows a good correlation with pulmonary vascular resistances [61]. VEC-MR is more efficient for the calculation of the pulmonary-to-sytemic flow ratio, so allowing non-invasive quantification of left-to-right shunts (see above) (Fig. 2.**29**) and evaluation of pulmonary pressure with various measurements derived from Doppler methods. These include estimation of maximum velocity in the jet of the usually associated tricuspid regurgitation on a four-chamber view and in the jet of a VSD on a sagittal oblique plane. By using the modified Bernoulli equation [$\Delta P = 4 \cdot (V_{max})^2$], where ΔP is the pressure gradient across the tricuspid valve and across the VSD respectively and V_{max} the peak velocity in m/sec measured in the regurgitant tricuspid jet and in the transventricular jet, respectively. Pulmonary pressure will be calculated as right atrial pressure (usually estimated to 10 mm Hg) + $4 \cdot (V_{max(tricuspid)})^2$. For a jet in a VSD, the systolic pulmonary pressure will be equal to the systolic aortic pressure (measured at the end of the examination) − $4 \cdot (V_{max(transventricular)})^2$ [62,63]. However, these methods have to be validated in large series of patients. Modifications of flow pattern in the main pulmonary artery have also been demonstrated in patients with pulmonary hypertension. Retrograde flow, usually negligible in normal subjects, accounted for one-fourth of the total flow in patients with pulmonary hypertension [54] and a significantly

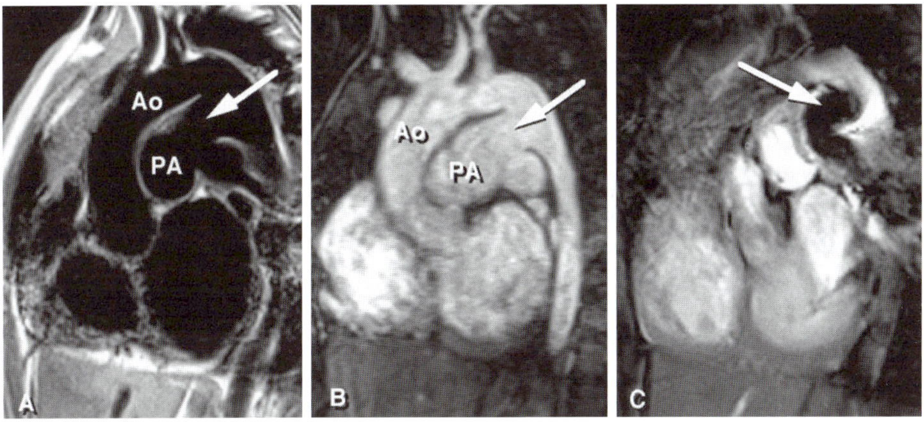

Fig. 2.**28**: Large patent ductus arteriosus (PDA) (arrow). The best imaging plane to demonstrate a PDA is the sagittal oblique view encompassing the aortic arch and the pulmonary bifurcation (**A**). Cine-GE images (**B**, **C**) help in showing the flow void due to a left-to-right shunt at this level on systolic images (arrow on **C**).

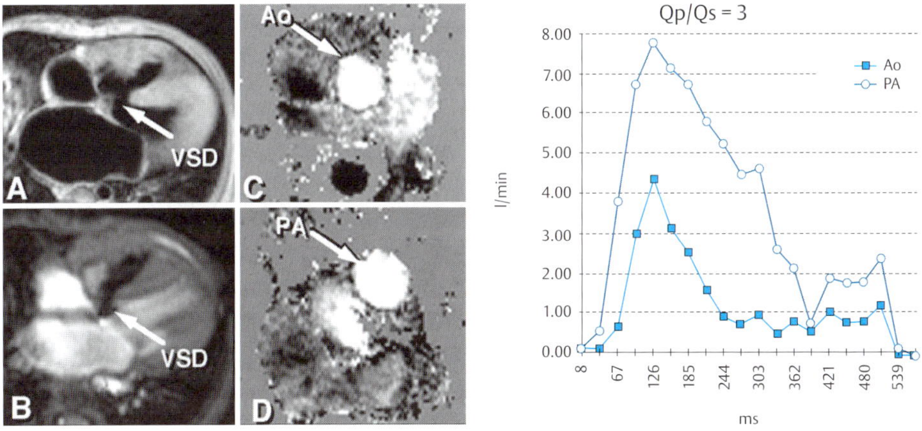

Fig. 2.**29** Transverse spin-echo (**A**), cine-GE (**B**) and velocity-encoded (VEC) phase images (**C**, **D**) at the level of pulmonary artery (PA) and ascending aorta (Ao) in a patient with a large perimembranous VSD and left-to-right shunt. VEC images allow the calculation of pulmonary and aortic flow. **E**: plot of aortic and pulmonary flow. Non-invasive quantification of pulmonary-to-systemic flow ratio (Qp/Qs) was calculated to be 3 in this case and was confirmed by oximetry.

lower peak systolic velocity was reached much earlier in systole in patients with pulmonary hypertension as compared to normal subjects [4,55].

Stenosis can occur as a solitary valvular lesion or as a component of a more complex disease at different levels of a cardiac chamber or a vascular structure. In all these cases the pressure gradient can be estimated non-invasively by VEC-MR with use of the modified Bernoulli equation [$\Delta P = 4 \cdot (V_{max})^2$] [16] (see Chapter 5 and fourth section of the companion CD-ROM). For valvular pulmonary stenosis, one of the therapeutic procedures is percutaneous valvuloplasty. Doppler echocardiography is the procedure of choice in evaluating the degree of pulmonary stenosis and is sufficient in the majority of cases to plan the therapeutic intervention. MRI can be useful in cases where the Doppler study is inconsistent with clinical data or insufficient, particularly when the acoustic window is limited. MRI, which displays the entire abnormal flow jet in any plane or direction, can provide a direct measurement of the degree of stenosis. Spin-echo images can demonstrate bulging of the pulmonary valve, right ventricular hypertrophy and poststenotic dilatation of the pulmonary artery at the level of the bifurcation. With the help of VEC-MR, the calculation of the maximum velocity (V_{max}) within the stenotic jet can be performed either on planes perpendicular or parallel to the direction of flow by using, respectively, slice select direction and frequency-encoded or phased-encoded direction sequences [33].

Evaluation of valvular stenosis and regurgitation is discussed in detail in the Chapter 5 and in the fourth section of the CD-ROM.

2.8 Other Miscellaneous Anomalies

2.8.1 Ebstein's Anomaly

Ebstein's anomaly is a rare malformation where the leaflets of the tricuspid valve are displaced toward the apex. The tricuspid annulus is in place but the leaflets did not separate normally from the right ventricular inflow tract. In the minor forms only the septal leaflet is involved. In severe forms the three leaflets may be attached distally. This results in the creation of an atrialized chamber between the right atrium and the remainder of the right ventricle, which realizes a functional obstruction to the filling of the right ventricle. The right atrium is markedly dilated and the left ventricle is compressed. Depending on the severity of the malformation there are four types of Ebstein's anomaly [66]. It is often associated with a secundum atrial septal defect. Pulmonary stenosis and ventricular septal defect may be associated as well. Ebstein's anomaly is frequently encountered on the tricuspid valve of a left-sided right ventricle in corrected transposition of the great arteries. The transverse and coronal planes are the most appropriate for defining the pathology (Fig. 2.**30**) [67].

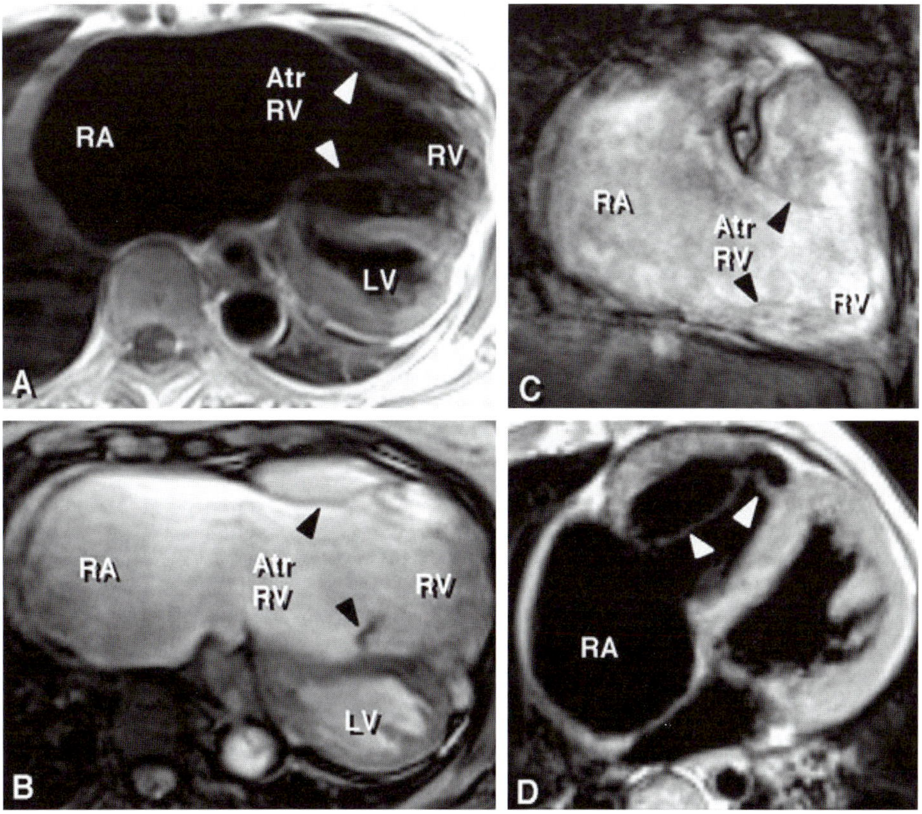

Fig. 2.**30** Ebstein's anomaly. Transverse (**A**, **B**) and coronal (**C**) spin-echo and cine-GE images in a severe form (type **C**) and minor form (type **A**) in another patient (**D**). In the severe form, the three leaflets of the tricuspid valve are displaced toward the apex and are attached distally (arrow-heads). It results the creation of an atrialized chamber (Atr RV) between the right atrium (RA) and the remainder of the right ventricle (RV) which realizes a functional obstruction to the filling of the right ventricle. The right atrium is markedly dilated and the left ventricle (LV) is compressed. In the minor form (**D**), only the septal leaflet is involved (arrow-heads).

2.8.2 Cor Triatriatum

Cor triatriatum is a rare malformation where there is a membrane within the left atrial cavity separating it into two portions: superior with pulmonary veins connection and inferior with the left atrial appendage and connecting with the mitral valve. This membrane is perforated and is responsible for obstruction of the pulmonary venous flow. The transverse and coronal planes are the most appropriate for defining the pathology (Fig. 2.**31**).

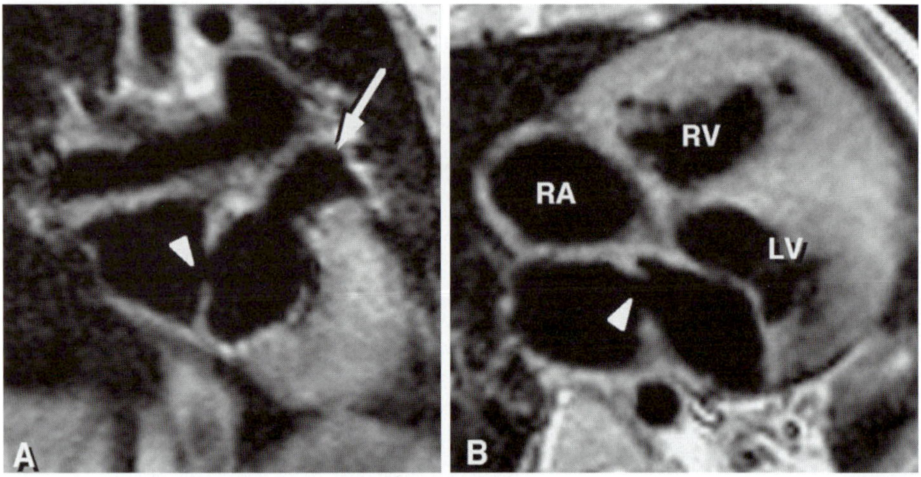

Fig. 2.**31** Cor triatriatum. Coronal (**A**) and transverse (**B**) spin-echo images. The perforated membrane (arrow-heads) within the left atrial cavity separating it into two portions: superior with pulmonary veins connection and inferior with the left atrial appendage (arrow) and connecting with the mitral valve, is well demonstrated.

2.9 Postoperative Evaluation of CHD in Adult Patients

During the recent years of development of cardiothoracic surgery, an increasingly large number of patients with CHD have been treated surgically (with both palliative and corrective surgery) and many of them have reached adulthood several years after surgery. The need for non-invasive procedures to follow-up these patients is crucial. Transthoracic two-dimensional and Doppler echocardiography may be limited by poor acoustic penetration due to scars, sternal wires, lung interposition and thoracic deformation due to the CHD resulting in poor image quality. MRI has proven its effectiveness in the evaluation and care of this growing population because the access to the chest is unlimited and because of its multi-oblique imaging capability. Different categories of patients may benefit from MRI: asymptomatic individuals after complete repair of their defect, symptomatic or asymptomatic patients with residual defects or complications of surgery and symptomatic patients who have had palliative procedures [10,11,12].

The role of MRI in the postoperative follow-up of thoracic aortic diseases such as coarctation of the aorta is treated in Chapter 3 and second section of the companion CD-ROM. Other situations where MRI is indicated are discussed below:

2.9.1 Patency and Complications in Systemic-to-Pulmonary Artery Shunts

Spin-echo imaging was recognized as a useful tool for identifying systemic-to-pulmonary artery shunts (see Fig. 2.**11**) but it is sometimes insufficient for demonstrating

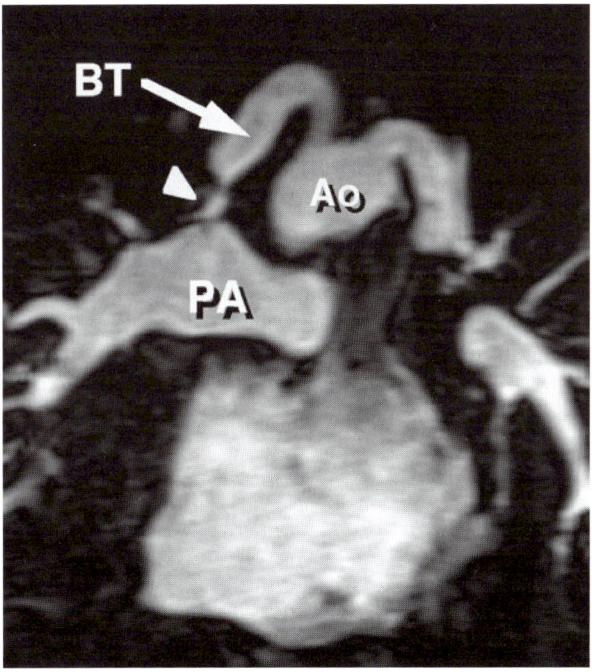

Fig. 2.**32** Coronal oblique multiplanar reconstruction of gadolinium-enhanced 3D MR angiography in a patient with pulmonary atresia and right and left Blalock-Taussig (BT) shunts. Due to its oblique course, the tight stenosis at the anastomosis of the right shunt (arrowhead) was not visualized on spin-echo images.

the entire shunt due to its oblique course. However, VEC MRI and MR angiographic techniques can help resolving these difficult diagnostic problems [68, 69] (Fig. 2.**32**).

2.9.2 Surgical Repair of Tetralogy of Fallot and Cono-Truncal Malformations

Total correction of tetralogy of Fallot includes reconstruction of the outflow tract with or without incorporation of a patch of pericardium or Dacron and closure of the VSD or, in severe forms, insertion of a homograft aortic valve or a conduit containing a prosthetic valve (Rastelli procedure) between the right ventricle and the pulmonary artery. MRI, using a combination of different imaging techniques, can be the most appropriate imaging modality in these cono-truncal malformations for demonstrating: residual stenosis, residual shunt, aneurysmal dilatation of reconstructed pulmonary outflow tract, degree of pulmonary regurgitation, stenosis, obstruction or pseudoaneurysm at the site of anastomosis of a conduit or a homograft. Evaluation of right ventricular function is important as well. Calculation of the regurgitant fraction can be monitored in order to plan the optimal timing for pulmonary valve replacement [5] (Figs. 2.**33** to 2.**37**).

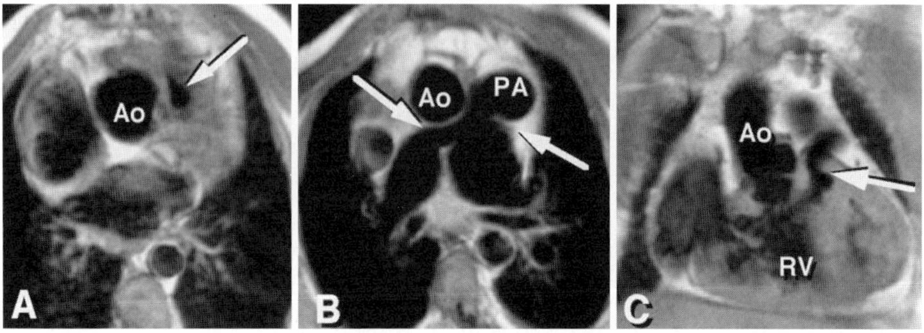

Fig. 2.**33** Status post repair of tetralogy of Fallot. Transverse (**A**, **B**) and coronal (**C**) images show a narrowing at the level of the outflow tract, the main pulmonary artery (PA) and the origin of the right pulmonary artery (arrows). Post-stenotic dilatation is visualized as well on pulmonary branches. Ao = aorta, RV = right ventricle.

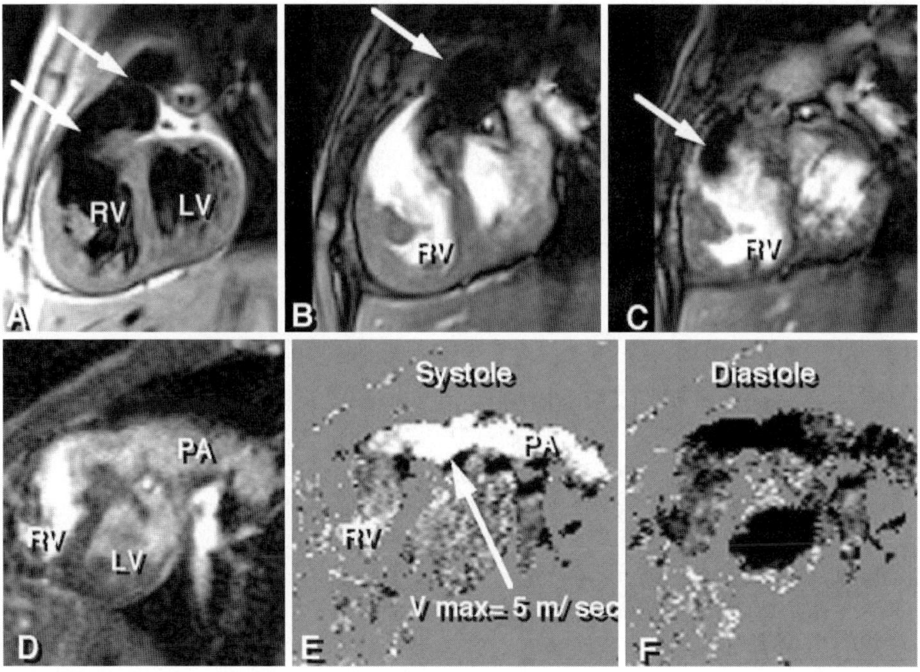

Fig. 2.**34** Status post repair of a tetralogy of Fallot. Sagittal spin-echo (**A**) and cine-GE images in systole (**B**) and in diastole (**C**) show a stenosis at the level of the outflow tract and the pulmonary valve (arrows). In systole (**B**), the signal void caused by high-velocity flow and turbulence extends far in the pulmonary artery suggesting a tight stenosis (arrow). In diastole (**C**), the retrograde signal void into the right ventricle (RV) suggests a severe pulmonary regurgitation (arrow). Magnitude (**D**) and phase (**E**, **F**) velocity-encoded images in systole (**E**) and in diastole (**F**) centered on the pulmonary artery (PA) allow one to calculate a maximum velocity of 5 m/second corresponding to a gradient of 100 mm Hg. Retrograde flow (in black on **F**) in diastole is well demonstrated as well.

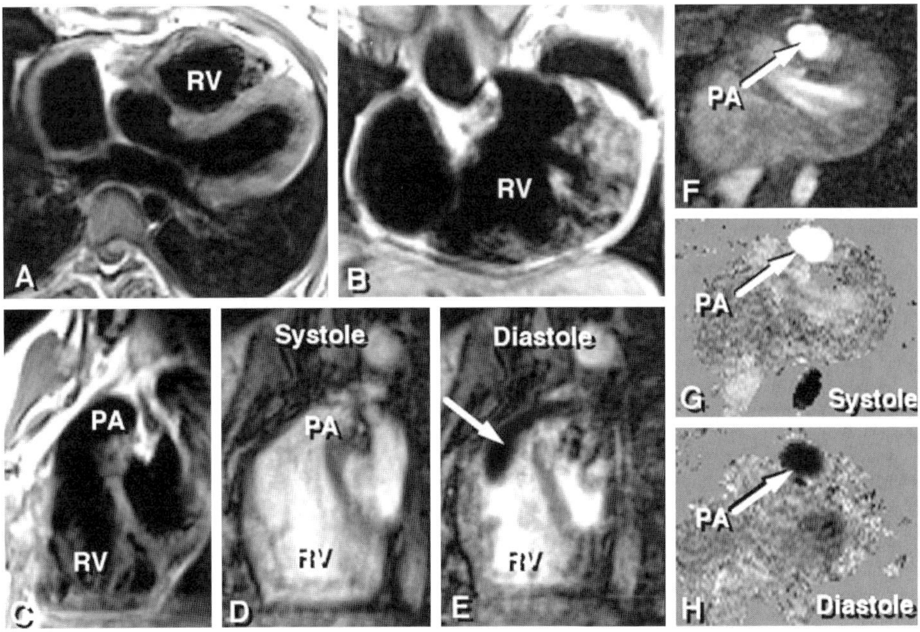

Fig. 2.**35** Status post repair of a tetralogy of Fallot. Spin-echo (**A**, **B**, **C**), and cine-GE (**D**, **E**) images show a dilatation of the right ventricle (RV) and the pulmonary artery (PA) and a retrograde signal void into the right ventricle (RV) suggesting a moderate pulmonary regurgitation (arrow on **E**). Magnitude (**F**) and phase (**G**, **H**) velocity-encoded images perpendicular to the pulmonary artery (PA). In systole, white coloration of the pixels within the PA indicates forward flow (**G**). In diastole, dark coloration of the pixels within the PA indicates retrograde flow (**H**). The pulmonary flow curve confirmed a moderate pulmonary regurgitation (regurgitation fraction of 33%).

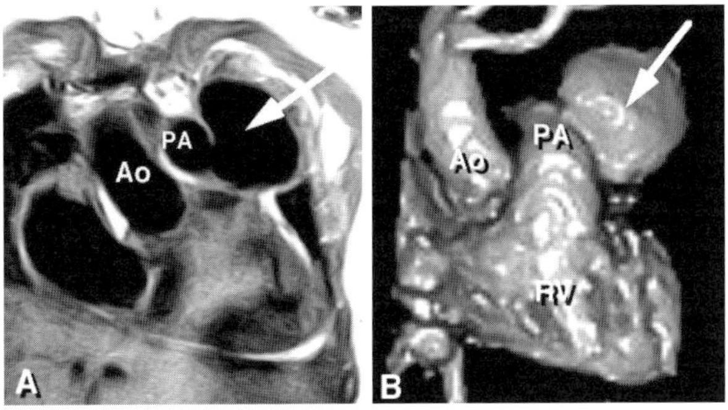

Fig. 2.**36** Status one year after complete correction of a type I truncus arteriosus with an aortic homograft positioned between the right ventricle (RV) and the pulmonary artery (PA). Spin-echo (**A**) and surface rendering of a gadolinium-enhanced MR angiography (**B**) demonstrate a false aneurysm at the anastomosis of the homograft and PA (arrow).

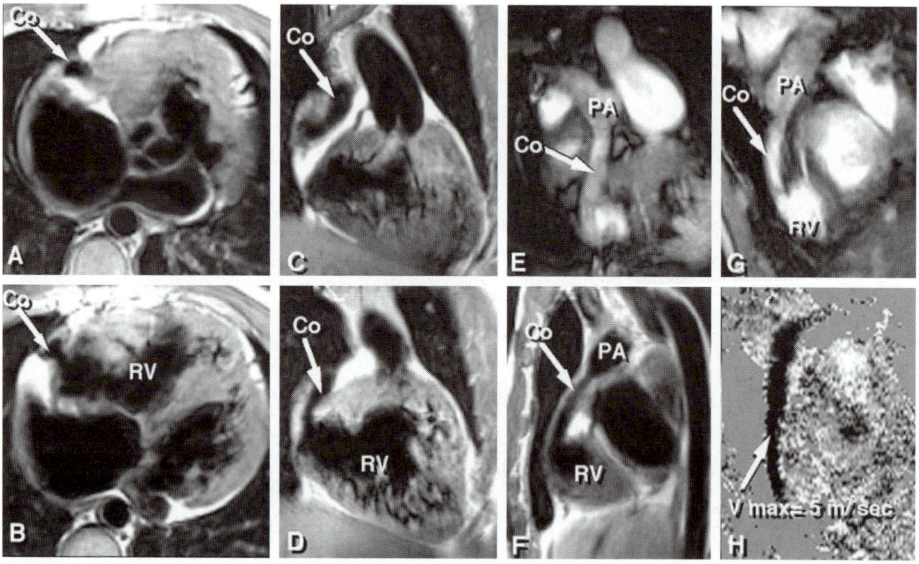

Fig. 2.**37** Patient with a double outlet left ventricle repaired with a Rastelli procedure [conduit (Co) between the right ventricle (RV) and the pulmonary artery (PA)]. The different images show a severe stenosis in the conduit, which was confirmed by the velocity-encoded images (**H**) with a maximum velocity of 5 m/second in the conduit corresponding to a gradient of 100 mm Hg.

2.9.3 Intracardiac Baffles and Patches

After Mustard or Senning operations for transposition of the great arteries the intra-atrial partitioning (Fig. 2.**38**) will be evaluated by spin-echo and cine-GE imaging to detect two types of complications: a residual shunt at the level of the baffle or the patch and obstruction of systemic and pulmonary venous pathways [70,71,72].

Fontan or modified Fontan operations and other cavopulmonary anastomoses result in a by-pass of the right heart in cases of tricuspid atresia or univentricular heart. It can be associated with an intracardiac baffle connecting a ventricular chamber to the aorta. Imaging will be directed to identify the connections of the inferior vena cava and the superior vena cava to the pulmonary arteries and the morphology of the intracardiac baffle in order to detect stenosis or obstruction at the level of anastomoses by spin-echo and cine-GE techniques [73]. VEC-MRI is the best method to determine the degree of stenosis. MR angiography is particularly suitable to show these venous anastomoses (Figs. 2.**39** and 2.**40**).

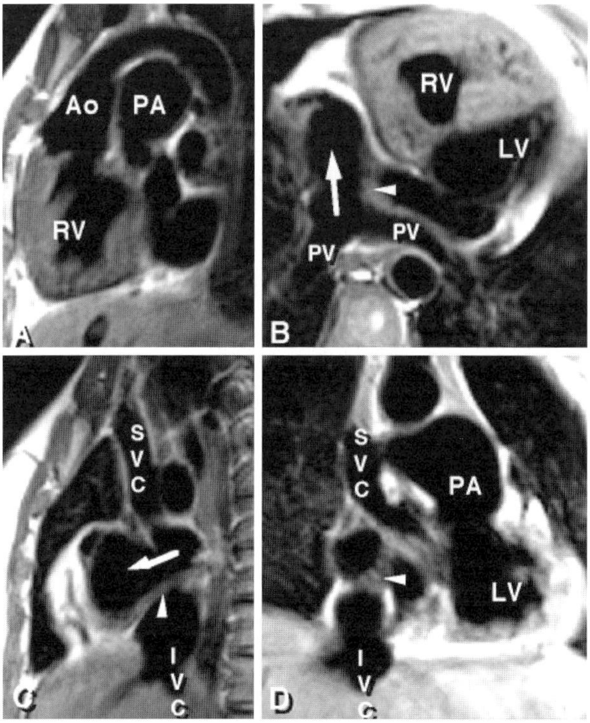

Fig. 2.**38** Patient with a D transposition of the great arteries repaired with a Mustard operation (atrial rerouting of venous blood flow). The intraatrial baffle (arrow-heads) rerouting the pulmonary veins (PV) towards the right atrium and the superior (SVC) and the inferior (IVC) vena cavae towards the left atrium (arrows) is well demonstrated. Note the aorta (Ao) arising from the hypertrophied right ventricle (RV).

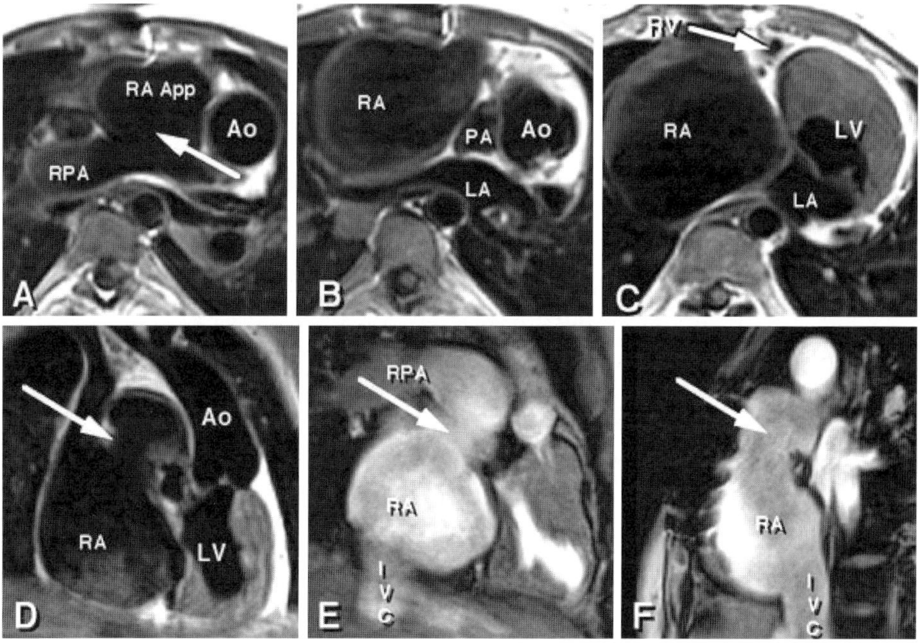

Fig. 2.**39** Patient with tricuspid atresia who underwent a Fontan procedure consisting of the connection of the right atrium (RA) at the level of the right atrial appendage (RA App) to the main pulmonary artery (PA) (arrow). Signal into the RA is due to slow blood flow. Note on **C** the high signal intensity in the right atrioventricular groove corresponding to the tricuspid atresia and the hypoplastic right ventricle (RV).

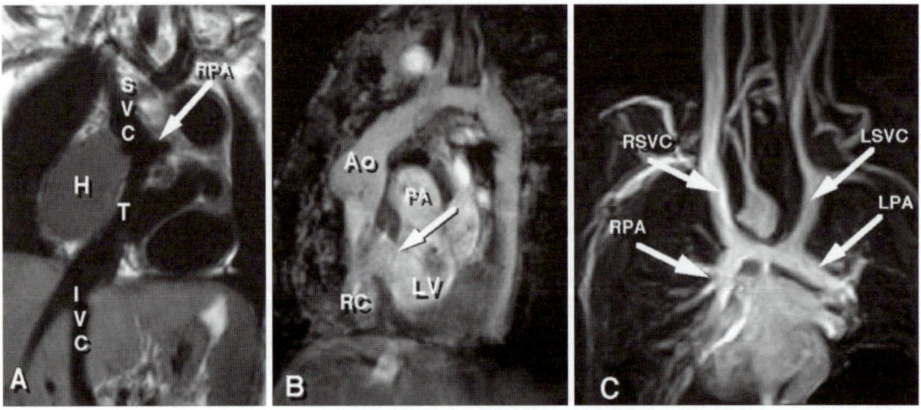

Fig. 2.**40** Two examples of by-pass of the right heart (modified Fontan operation). In **A** and **B**, coronal spin-echo (**A**) and sagittal cine-GE (**B**) images of a patient with type A single ventricle, L malposition of the great vessels and single atrioventricular valve. The main chamber is a left ventricular (LV) type chamber. The rudimentary chamber (RC) is located anterosuperiorly and was connected to the aorta (Ao), anterior and to the left of the pulmonary artery (PA). The procedure consisted of complete banding of the PA trunk, intracardiac baffle connecting the main chamber to the aorta (arrow) and lateral tunnel (T) connecting the inferior vena cava (IVC) to the superior vena cava (SVC) and the pulmonary arteries branches (RPA). A postoperative pericardial hematoma is visualized as an area of medium signal intensity (H). In **C**, MIP reconstruction of a 3D breath-hold gadolinium-enhanced MR angiography in a patient with severe tetralogy of Fallot and atrioventricular canal after double anastomosis of right and left superior vena cava to the right and left pulmonary arteries (arrows).

2.9.4 Arterial Switch Operation for Transposition of the Great Vessels

The arterial switch operation consists of transection of the great arteries and direct reanastomosis of the distal aortic segment to the proximal pulmonary artery and the distal pulmonary segment to the proximal aortic segment with transfer of the coronary artery ostia to the pulmonary root. Thus, the ascending aorta is positioned posteriorly to the main pulmonary artery. MRI is the best technique for detecting the complications after this surgical procedure, particularly the stenosis of pulmonary artery branches (Fig. 2.**41**) and of supravalvular pulmonary arterial region, obstruction of the right ventricular outflow tract and bronchial compression [7].

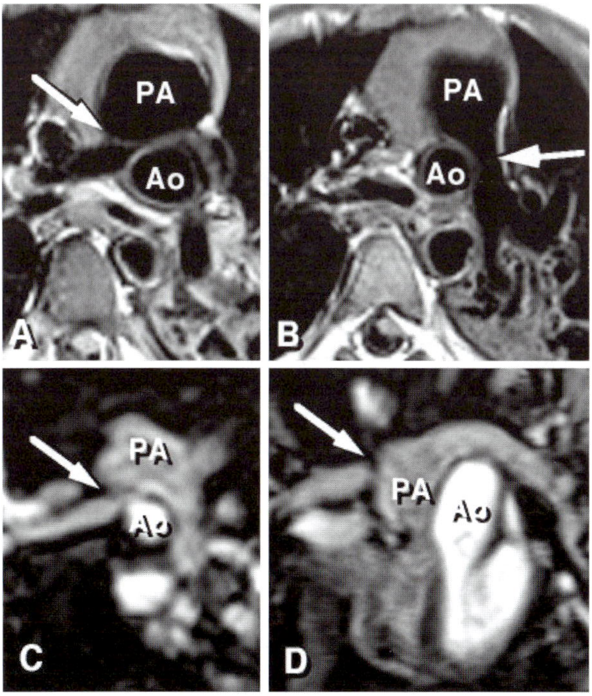

Fig. 2.**41** Patient with D transposition of the great arteries who underwent an arterial switch operation (Jatene procedure). Transverse spin-echo (**A**, **B**) and oblique multiplanar reconstructions of a gadolinium-enhanced 3D MR angiography (**C**, **D**) demonstrate a slight narrowing of the left pulmonary artery (arrow on **B**) and a more severe stenosis at the origin of the right pulmonary artery (arrow on **A**, **C**, **D**).

2.10 References

1. Higgins CB, Byrd BF III, Farmer DW, et al. Magnetic resonance imaging in patients with congenital heart disease. Circulation 1984; 70: 851–860.
2. Didier D, Higgins CB, Fisher MR, et al. Gated magnetic resonance imaging in congenital heart disease: experience in initial 72 patients. Radiology 1986; 158: 227–235.
3. Didier D, Ratib O, Beghetti M, et al. Morphologic and functional evaluation of congenital heart disease by magnetic resonance imaging. J Magn Reson Imaging 1999; 10: 639–655.
4. Fletcher BD, Jacobstein MD, Nelson AD, et al. Gated magnetic resonance imaging of congenital cardiac malformations. Radiology 1984; 150: 137–140.
5. Rebergen SA, Niezen RA, Helbing WA, van der Wall EE, de Roos A. Cine gradient echo MR imaging and MR velocity mapping in the evaluation of congenital heart disease. RadioGraphics 1996; 16: 467–481.
6. Szolar DH, Sakuma H, Higgins CB. Cardiovascular applications of magnetic resonance flow and velocity measurements. JMRI 1996; 1: 78–89.
7. Higgins CB, Silvermann NH, Kersting-Sommerhoff BA, Schmid TK. Congenital heart disease. In: Echocardiography and Magnetic Resonance Imaging. Raven Press, New York, 1990.

8. Fletcher BD, Jacobstein MD. MRI of congenital abnormalities of the great arteries. AJR 1986; 146: 941–948.
9. Higgins CB. The Heart: Congenital disease. In: Magnetic resonance imaging of the body. Raven Press, New York, 1992; 267–293.
10. Gross GW, Steiner RM. Radiographic manifestations of congenital heart disease in the adult patient. Radiol Clin North America 1991; 29: 293–317.
11. Wexler L, Higgins CB. The use of magnetic resonance imaging in adult congenital heart disease. Am J Card Imaging 1995; 9: 15–28.
12. Hoppe UC, Dederichs B, Deutsch HJ, et al. Congenital heart disease in adults and adolescents. Comparative value of transthoracic and transesophageal echocardiography and MR imaging. Radiology 1996; 199: 669–677.
13. Underwood SR, Firmin DN, Klipstein RH, Rees RSO, Longmore DB. Magnetic resonance velocity mapping: Clinical application of a new technique. Br Heart J 1987; 57: 404–412.
14. Nayler GL, Firmin DN, Longmore DB. Blood flow imaging by cine magnetic resonance. J Comput Assist Tomography 1987; 10: 715–722.
15. Rees S, Firmin DN, Mohiaddin R, et al. Application of flow measurements by magnetic resonance to congenital heart disease. Am J Cardiol 1989; 64: 953–956.
16. Mostbeck GH, Caputo GR, Higgins CB. MR measurements of blood flow in the cardiovascular system. AJR 1992; 159: 453–461.
17. Rebergen SA, van der Wall EE, Doornbos J, et al. Magnetic resonance measurements of velocity and flow: Technique, validation and cardiovascular applications. Am Heart J 1993; 126:1439–1456.
18. Ho VB, Prince MR. Thoracic MR aortography: Imaging techniques and strategies. RadioGraphics 1998; 18: 287–309.
19. Krinsky GA, Rofsky NM, DeCorato DR, et al. Thoracic aorta: comparison of gadolinium-enhanced three-dimensional MR angiography and conventional MR imaging. Radiology 1997; 202: 183–193.
20. Didier D, Ratib O, Lerch R, Friedli B. Detection and quantification of valvular heart disease with dynamic cardiac MR imaging. RadioGraphics 2000; 20: 1279–1299.
21. Task Force of the European Society of Cardiology, in collaboration with the Association of European Paediatric Cardiologists. The clinical role of magnetic resonance in cardiovascular disease. Eur Heart J 1998; 19: 19–39.
22. Boxt LM. MR imaging of congenital heart disease. MRI Clin of North America 1996; 4: 327–359.
23. Choe YH, Kim YM, Han BK, et al. MR imaging of the morphologic diagnosis of congenital heart disease. RadioGraphics 1997; 17: 403–422.
24. Kondo C, Caputo GR, Semelka R, et al. Right and left ventricular stroke volume measurements with velocity-encoded cine MR imaging: In vitro and in vivo validation. AJR 1991; 157: 9–16.
25. Sechtem U, Pflugfelder PW, White RD, et al. Cine MR imaging: Potential for the evaluation of cardiovascular function. AJR 1987; 148: 239–246.

26. Simpson IA, Chung KJ, Glass RF, et al. Cine magnetic resonance imaging for evaluation of anatomy and flow relations in infants and children with coarctation of the aorta. Circulation 1988; 78: 142–148.
27. Didier D, Ratib O, Friedli B, et al. Cine gradient-echo MR imaging in the evaluation of cardiovascular diseases. RadioGraphics 1993; 13: 561–573.
28. Suzuki JI, Caputo GR, Kondo C, Higgins CB. Cine MR imaging of valvular heart disease: display and imaging parameters affect the size of the signal void caused by valvular regurgitation. AJR 1990; 155: 723–727.
29. Baldy C, Doueck P, Croisille P, et al. Automated myocardial edge detection from breath-hold cine-MR images: Evaluation of left ventricular volumes and mass. Magn Reson Imaging 1994; 12: 589–592.
30. Higgins CB, Sakuma H. Heart disease: Functional evaluation with MR imaging. Radiology 1996; 199: 307–315.
31. Firmin D, Underwood R. Magnetic resonance flow imaging. In: Magnetic Resonance of the Cardiovascular System. Underwood R, Firmin D (eds), Blackwell Scientific Publications, Oxford, 1991.
32. Firmin DN, Nayler GL, Kipstein RH, et al. In vivo validation of MR velocity imaging. J Comput Assist Tomography 1987; 11: 751–756.
33. Higgins CB, Caputo G, Wendland MF, Saeed M. Measurement of blood flow and perfusion in the cardiovascular system. Invest Radiol 1992; 27: S66–S71.
34. Mohiaddin RH, Pennell DJ. MR blood flow measurement. Clinical application in the heart and circulation. Cardiol Clin 1998; 16: 161–187.
35. Brenner LD, Caputo GR, Mostbeck G, et al. Quantification of left to right atrial shunts with velocity-encoded cine nuclear magnetic resonance imaging. J Am Coll Cardiol 1992; 20: 1246–1250.
36. Hundley WG, Li HF, Lange RA, et al. Assessment of left-to-right intracardiac shunting by velocity-encoded, phase-difference magnetic resonance imaging. A comparison with oximetric and indicator dilution techniques. Circulation 1995; 91: 2955–2960.
37. Caputo GR, Kondo C, Masui T, et al. Right and left lung perfusion: in vitro and in vivo validation with oblique-angle, velocity-encoded cine MR imaging. Radiology 1991; 180: 693–698.
38. Bogren HG, Buonocore MH. Blood flow measurements in the aorta and major arteries with MR velocity mapping. JMRI 1994; 4: 119–130.
39. Kilner PJ, Manzara CC, Mohiaddin RH, et al. Magnetic resonance jet velocity mapping in mitral and aortic valve stenosis. Circulation 1993; 87: 1239–1248.
40. Van Praagh R. Terminology of congenital disease. Glossary and commentary. Circulation 1977; 56: 139–143.
41. Van Praagh R, Weinberg PW, Van Praagh S. Malpositions of the heart. In: Heart Disease in Infants, Children and Adolescents. Moss AF, Adams FH, Emmanouilides GC (eds), Williams and Wilkins, Baltimore, 1977.
42. Akins EW, Martin TD, Alexander JA, et al. MR imaging of double outlet right ventricle. AJR 1989; 152: 128–130.

43. Rees RS, Somerville J, Underwood SR, et al. Magnetic resonance imaging of the pulmonary arteries and their systemic connections in pulmonary atresia: comparison with angiographic and surgical findings. Br Heart J 1987; 58: 621–626.
44. Mirovitz SA, Gutierrez FR, Canter CE, et al. Tetralogy of Fallot. MR findings. Radiology 1989; 171: 207–212.
45. Kersting-Sommerhoff BA, Sechtem UP, Higgins CB. Evaluation of blood supply by nuclear magnetic resonance imaging in patients with pulmonary atresia. J Am Coll Cardiology 1988; 11: 166–171.
46. Soulen RL, Donner RM, Capitanio M. Postoperative evaluation of complex congenital heart disease by MRI. RadioGraphics 1987; 7: 975–1000.
47. Donnelly LF, Higgins CB. MR imaging of conotruncal abnormalities. AJR 1996; 166: 925–928.
48. Van Praagh R, Van Praagh S, Nebesar RA, et al. Tetralogy of Fallot: Underdevelopment of the pulmonary infundibulum and its sequealae. Am J Cardiology 1970; 26: 25–33.
49. Formanek AG, Witcofski RL, D'Souza VJ, et al. MR imaging of the central pulmonary arterial tree in cono-truncal malformation. AJR 1986; 147: 1127–1131.
50. Van Praagh R, Van Praagh S. The anatomy of common aortico-pulmonary trunk (truncus arteriosus communis) and its embryologic implications. A study of 57 recropsied cases. Am J Cardiology 1965; 16: 406–425.
51. Van Praagh R, Ongley PA, Swan HJC. Anatomic types of single or common ventricule in man. Morphologic and geometric aspects of sixty autopsied cases. Am J Cardiology 1964; 13: 367–386.
52. Jacobstein MD, Portman MA, Fletcher BD. Magnetic resonance imaging in uni-ventricular atrioventricular connection. Am J Card Imaging 1987; 1: 221–226.
53. Anderson RH, Becker AS, Macartney FJ, et al. Is tricuspid atresia a univentricular heart. Pediatr Cardiol 1979; 1: 51–56.
54. Masui T, Seelos KC, Kersting-Sommerhoff BA, et al. Abnormalities of the pulmonary veins: evaluation with MR imaging and comparison with cardiac angiography and echocardiography. Radiology 1991; 181: 645–649.
55. Dinsmore RE, Eesmir GL, Guyer D, et al. Magnetic resonance imaging of the interatrial septum and atrial septal defect. AJR 1985; 145: 697–703.
56. Diethelm L, Dery R, Lipton MJ, Higgins CB. Sensitivity and specificity of magnetic resonance for identification and localization of atrial level shunts. Radiology 1987; 162: 181–186.
57. Lowell DG, Turner DH, Smith SM, et al. The detection of atrial and ventricular septal defects with EGG synchronised magnetic resonance imaging. Circulation 1986; 73: 89–94.
58. Didier D, Higgins CB. Identification and localization of ventricular septal defects by gated magnetic resonance imaging. Am J Cardiology 1986; 57: 1363–1368.
59. Jacobstein MD, Fletcher BD, Golstein S, et al. Evaluation of atrioventricular septal defect by magnetic resonance imaging. Am J Cardiol 1985; 55: 1158–1161.

60. Sechtem U, Pflugfelder P, Cassidy MC, et al. Ventricular septal defect: Visualization of shunt flow and determination of shunt size by cine magnetic resonance imaging. AJR 1987; 149: 689–692.
61. Didier D, Higgins CB. Estimation of pulmonary vascular resistance by MRI in patients with congenital cardiovascular lesions. AJR 1986; 146: 919–924.
62. Yock PG, Popp RL. Non-invasive estimation of right ventricular systolic pressure by Doppler ultrasound in patients with tricuspid regurgitation. Circulation 1984; 70: 657–662.
63. Murphy DJ, Ludomirsky A, Hunta JC. Continuous-wave Doppler in children with ventricular septal defect: non-invasive estimation of intraventricular pressure gradient. Am J Cardiol 1986; 57: 428–432.
64. Bogren HG, Klipstein RH, Mohiaddin RH, et al. Pulmonary artery distensibility and blood flow patterns: a magnetic resonance study of normal subjects and of patients with pulmonary arterial hypertension. Am Heart J 1990; 118: 990–999.
65. Kondo C, Caputo GR, Masui T, et al. Pulmonary hypertension: pulmonary flow quantification and flow profile analysis with velocity-encoded cine MR imaging. Radiology 1992; 183: 751–758.
66. Carpentier A, Chauvaud S, Mace L, et al. A new reconstructive operation for Ebstein's anomaly of the tricuspid valve. J Thorac Cardiovasc Surg 1988; 96: 91–101.
67. Link KM, Herrera MA, D'Suoza VJ, Formanek AG. MR imaging of Ebstein's anomaly: results in four cases. Am J Roentgenol 1988; 150: 363–367.
68. Jacobstein MD, Fletcher BD, Nelson AD, et al. Magnetic resonance imaging: evaluation of palliative systemic pulmonary artery shunts. Circulation 1984; 70: 650–656.
69. Duerinckx A, Atkinson D, Klitzner TS, et al. MR imaging of surgical complications of systemic-to-pulmonary artery shunts. Magn Reson Imaging 1996; 14: 1099–1105.
70. Campbell RM, Moreau GA, Johns JA, et al. Detection of caval obstruction by MRI after intraatrial repair of transposition of great arteries. Am J Cardiol 1987; 60: 688–691.
71. Chung KJ, Simpson IA, Glass RF, et al. Cine MR after surgical repair in patients with transposition of great arteries. Circulation 1988; 77: 104–109.
72. Kersting-Sommerhoff BA, Seelos KC, Hardy C, et al. Evaluation of surgical procedures for cyanotic congenital heart disease by using MR imaging. AJR 1990; 155: 259.
73. Weinberg PM, Fogel MA. Cardiac imaging in congenital heart disease. Cardiol Clinics 1998; 16: 315–348.

3 Thoracic Aorta

Magnetic resonance imaging (MRI) is widely recognized as the non-invasive technique of choice in the pre- and postoperative assessment of thoracic aortic congenital and acquired diseases [1–5]. Unlike CT and conventional angiographies, the method is non-invasive and is capable of depicting, without the need for contrast media, the perivascular and vascular structures and with the help of velocity-encoded technique enables a quantitative assessment of associated flow anomalies [6]. MRI has several advantages in the assessment of the great arteries of the thorax over echocardiography, which is limited by a poor acoustic window, particularly in adult patients as well as in patients post surgical interventions [7].

Three-dimensional (3D) gadolinium-enhanced MR angiography (MRA) has recently been recommended by several authors for the evaluation of the thoracic aorta in congenital and acquired anomalies [8,9]. It has replaced time-of-flight and phase-contrast MR angiography techniques that are subject to artifacts from turbulent and abnormal blood flow [10]. This new technique, relying on the T1 shortening of blood flow by gadolinium contrast media in the circulation, which eliminates the flow artifacts seen with other methods, has evolved very quickly with higher resolution and shorter acquisition time. Moreover, this method provides volumetric data that may be processed for multiple reconstruction techniques including maximum intensity projection (MIP), curved multiplanar reformation (MPR) and surface and volume rendering [11].

This chapter describes the role of the different types of MR imaging techniques in the pre- and postoperative evaluation of aortic diseases with emphasis on MR angiography. For the description of the different imaging techniques, see the first and the second chapters and for examples of dynamic images of selected aortic anomalies, see the second section in the companion CD-ROM.

3.1 Coarctation of the Aorta

Coarctation of the aorta is a congenital stenosis commonly located in the region of the ductus arteriosus at the junction of the aortic arch and descending aorta (aortic isthmus) just distal to the left subclavian artery. MRI is the method of choice for the preoperative evaluation of coarctation of the aorta demonstrating all the parameters necessary to plan the surgical or interventional repair. The site, the degree of the stenosis as well as the length of the narrowing are precisely defined with MR imaging sequences. The degree of associated aortic arch tubular hypoplasia, the collateral pathways (internal mammary and posterior mediastinal arteries), the poststenotic

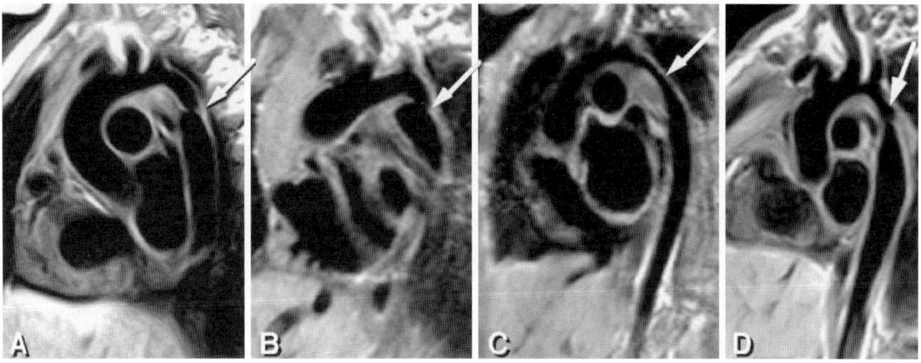

Fig. 3.**1** Oblique sagittal spin-echo images in different types of coarctation (arrows). Severe focal narrowing with shelf-like deformity is demonstrated at the junction between the aortic arch and the descending aorta in **A**. In **B**, only a portion of the aorta is displayed on the sagittal image due to aortic deformity and tortuous course of the vessel. The isthmal narrowing is immediately followed by a poststenotic dilatation. Long segment isthmal tubular hypoplasia is shown in **C**. Association of focal narrowing, poststenotic dilatation and moderate tubular hypoplasia of the distal aortic arch is shown in **D**.

dilatation, the relationship to the left subclavian artery and the degree of left ventricular hypertrophy are also well defined with MRI [12–15].

Transverse spin-echo images at the level of the aortic arch and the isthmus allow definition of the oblique plane of the aorta in the thorax and may identify the narrowing but this is very often obscured by a partial volume effect. The entire thoracic aorta is usually optimally visualized on oblique sagittal images. The coarctation appears as a focal shelf-like deformity associated or not with a long segment tubular hypoplasia of the isthmus depending upon the degree and the length of the narrowing (Fig. 3.**1**). But in many cases it cannot be demonstrated on a single plane because of the displacement of a portion of the thoracic aorta due to the coarctation and aortic tortuosity very common in this malformation [3]. The coronal plane encompassing the origin of descending aorta may help in numerous cases in showing the aortic narrowing (Fig. 3.**2**).

Cine-GE oblique sagittal images should be acquired systematically after spin-echo imaging. On cine-GE images, the narrowing corresponding to the coarctation will be evaluated on diastolic images. A signal void due to high-velocity turbulent flow across the coarctation, resulting in spin dephasing is depicted on systolic images. The severity of the narrowing can be qualitatively assessed by showing the size and the length of this signal void immediately distal to the coarctation [16] (Fig. 3.**3**). The tortuous course of the aorta may be a problem as well with this technique. Acquisition of several adjacent oblique sagittal planes with partial overlap, subsequently reconstructed with the maximum intensity projection algorithm (MIP), solves this problem [16]. The resulting image corresponding to the sum of the adjacent planes can be shown in a cine loop as a standard cine allowing the display of the entire thickness of

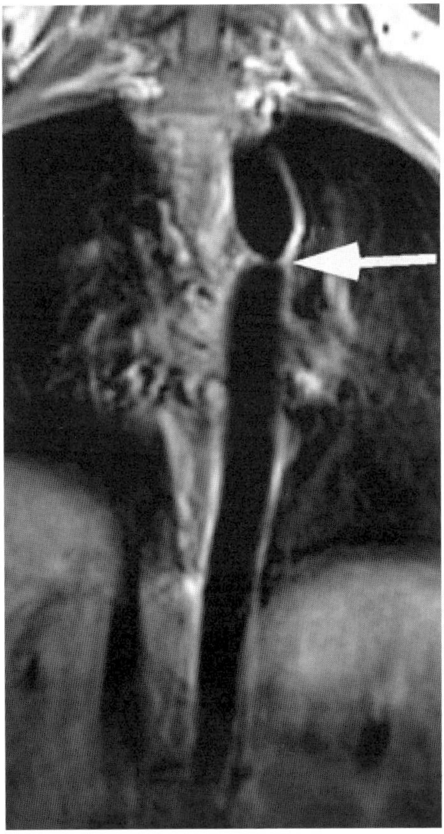

Fig. 3.**2** Coronal spin-echo image of the same patient as in Fig. 3.**1B**. The focal narrowing with shelf-like deformity is better demonstrated on this plane than in the oblique sagittal image (arrow).

the vessel with an added volume effect whereas the flow information provided by the individual planar cine sequences is maintained (Fig. 3.**4**).

For precise quantification of the pressure gradient across the coarctation, the velocity-encoded cine MR technique (VEC) allows one to measure directly the increased flow velocity within the stenotic jet demonstrated on cine-GE images [17,18]. The calculation of the peak velocity or maximum velocity (V_{max}) within the stenotic jet can be performed either on planes perpendicular to the direction of flow (through-plane velocity measurement) (transverse images) or parallel to the direction of flow (in-plane velocity measurement). Sagittal and coronal planes parallel to the direction of flow, encompassing the length of the jet, with velocity encoded vertically are optimal for this measurement [19] (Fig. 3.**5**). In-plane imaging yields numerous pixels for analysis of velocity because the entire abnormal jet is displayed. But in cases of very tight stenosis, where the jet is narrowed, in-plane measurement may be less reliable because of partial volume averaging and motion of the jet out of the imaging plane. Conversely, with through-plane imaging, only a slice of the jet is displayed and one can miss the maximum velocity if the plane is positioned too far from or too close

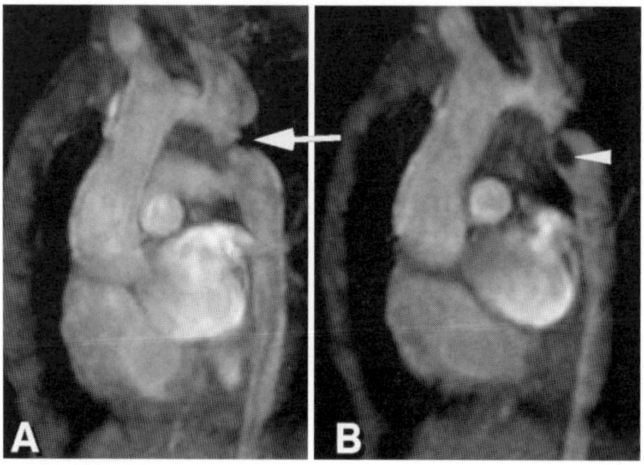

Fig. 3.**3** Oblique sagittal cine-GE images in diastole (**A**) and systole (**B**) of a patient with a tight coarctation. The focal narrowing just distal to the left subclavian artery is well demonstrated on the diastolic image (arrow). On the systolic image, a flow void (arrow-head) emanating from the narrowing and propagating in the descending aorta corresponds to high-velocity turbulent flow.

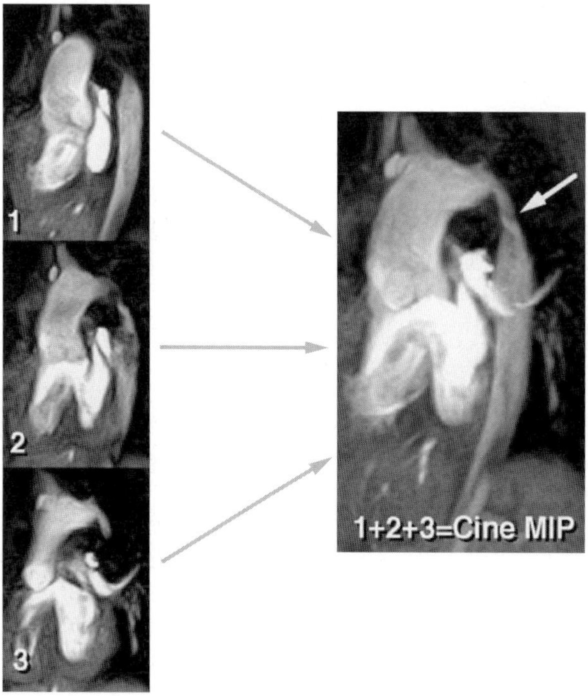

Fig. 3.**4** Oblique sagittal cine-GE images of a patient with a long segment coarctation and tubular isthmal hypoplasia. Three adjacent planes with partial overlap (1, 2, 3) were performed but the entire aorta could not be shown adequately on any of these projections due to the tortuous course of the vessel. A subsequent reconstruction of these three planes with the maximum intensity projection algorithm (cine-MIP) permitted us to image the entire thoracic aorta and particularly the narrowed isthmal segment.

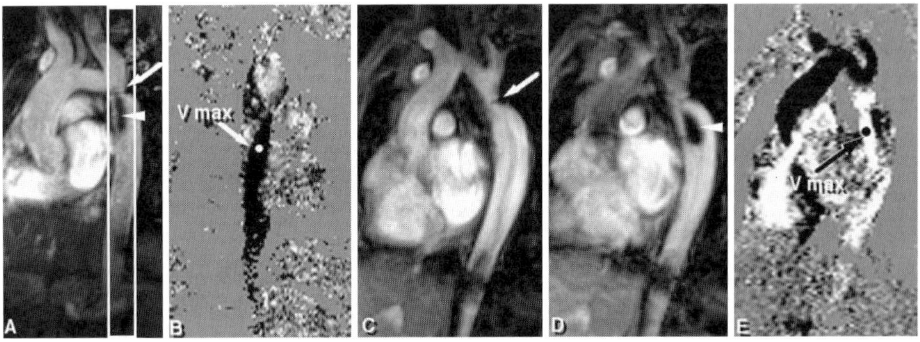

Fig. 3.**5** Cine-GE and velocity-encoded cine (VEC) MR images in two different patients with a tight coarctation. The stenosis is well demonstrated on sagittal cine-GE images (arrows) (**A**, **C**, **D**) as well as the flow void corresponding to high velocity flow emanating from the stenosis (arrow-heads). The calculation of the peak velocity or maximum velocity (V_{max}) within the stenotic jet was performed on coronal (**B**) and sagittal (**E**) planes parallel to the direction of flow, encompassing the length of the jet, with velocity encoded vertically (in-plane velocity measurement). A region of interest (black and white dots) was positioned within the jet. It allows the measurement of a V_{max} of 3.8 m/sec (**A**, **B**) and 4 m/sec (**C**, **D**) corresponding to a gradient of 58 mm Hg and 64 mm Hg, respectively, by using modified Bernoulli equation.

to the origin of the narrowing. Furthermore, misregistration of flow due to signal loss depending upon turbulence and eddy currents may occur if the plane is too close to the origin of the stenosis. Thus, it is preferable to measure data in both in- and through-planes [20]. Practically, because of the short acquisition time of these sequences, two in-plane velocity measurements (oblique sagittal and coronal) and one or several through-plane velocity measurements (transverse images below the coarctation) can be performed. The calculation of V_{max} is usually easy for velocities less than 4 m/sec but for velocities up to 6 m/sec the use of short TE sequence (TE = 3–4 ms) is mandatory to improve the reliability and accuracy of the measurements [20].

The pressure gradient (ΔP) across the narrowing can be derived using the modified Bernoulli equation, $\Delta P = 4 \cdot (V_{max})^2$ where ΔP is the pressure drop across the stenosis and V_{max} the peak velocity in m/sec measured in the stenotic jet (Fig. 3.**5**). Estimation of collateral circulation can be carried out as well with VEC-MR by measuring flow in the proximal and distal parts of the descending aorta. In hemodynamically significant coarctation there is an increase in flow in the distal compared with the proximal part of the descending aorta due to the collateral flow coming from the intercostal arteries. Collateral flow will be calculated as flow in the distal descending aorta minus flow in the proximal descending aorta [21].

3D gadolinium-enhanced MR angiography is at present the alternative or complementary technique to cine-GE sequence to image the entire thoracic aorta. It has been proven to be particularly valuable in diagnosing accurately congenital anomalies such as coarctation of the aorta [8, 9]. Initial experience was made by using non-breath-hold techniques, which provided high-quality projections, but respiratory motion

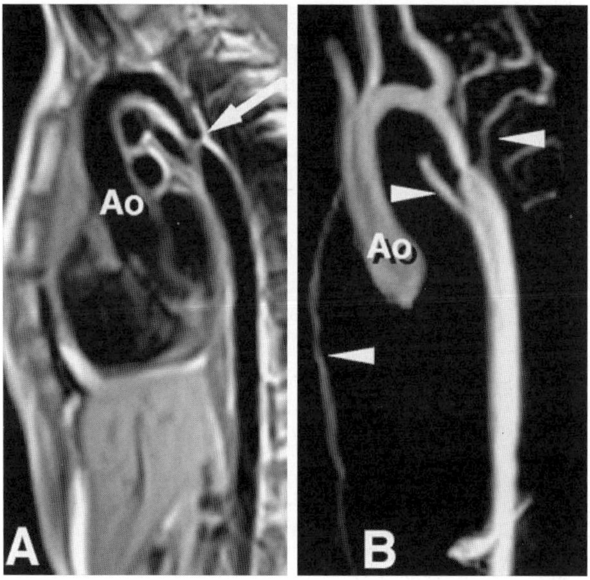

Fig. 3.**6** Oblique sagittal spin-echo image (**A**) and MIP reconstruction of a contrast-enhanced MR angiography (**B**) in a three-year-old girl with a tight coarctation associated with a long segment hypoplasia of the aortic arch (arrow). Numerous collaterals are particularly well demonstrated on MR angiography (arrow-heads).

degrades the quality of images of the intrathoracic great vessels. Recently, the use of breath-hold techniques with short TR and TE allows one to minimize respiration-induced motion artifacts and to reduce acquisition time [22]. These MR angiography techniques are non-invasive and provide cross-sectional data including intraluminal as well as extraluminal components of the vascular disease, thus yielding a unique information. The source images obtained by this technique must be analyzed on a computer workstation console and can be further reconstructed using different rendering and reformatting techniques, the most frequently used being maximum intensity projection (MIP) algorithm which provides an image similar to conventional contrast X-ray angiography (Fig. 3.**6**). However, this reconstruction technique has limitations such as overestimation of aortic narrowing. In some cases, the source images can be first segmented to remove superimpositions of undesirable other vascular and anatomic structures and to minimize wrap-around artifacts (aliasing).

The other reconstruction techniques such as multiplanar reformation (MPR) and 3D surface rendering (SR) or volume rendering (VR) can also be used (Fig. 3.**7**). Curved MPR in the plane of the aortic arch and after "elongation" of the entire thoracic aorta are the best techniques for accurate measurement of aortic dimensions and evaluation the degree of vascular narrowing (see section 2 of the CD-ROM).

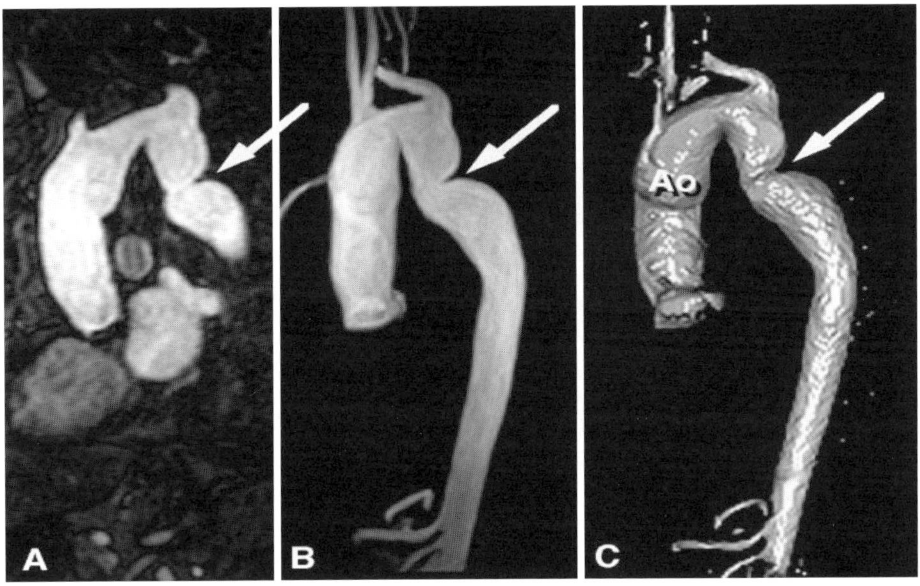

Fig. 3.**7** Source (**A**), MIP (**B**) and surface rendering (**C**) images of a 3D gadolinium-enhanced MR angiography of a moderate coarctation (arrows) associated with poststenotic dilatation of the proximal descending aorta.

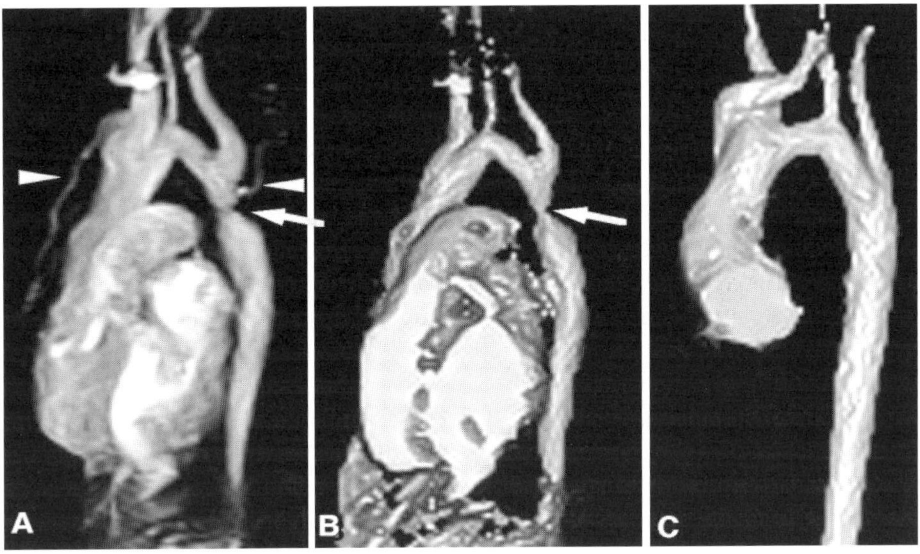

Fig. 3.**8** Tight coarctation. MIP (**A**) and surface rendering (**B**, **C**) of a 3D gadolinium-enhanced MR angiography before (**A**, **B**) and after resection and end-to-end anastomosis (**C**). Preoperative images show the severe narrowing (arrows) and the collaterals (arrow-heads). Postoperative study demonstrates a good result but persistence of moderate aortic arch hypoplasia.

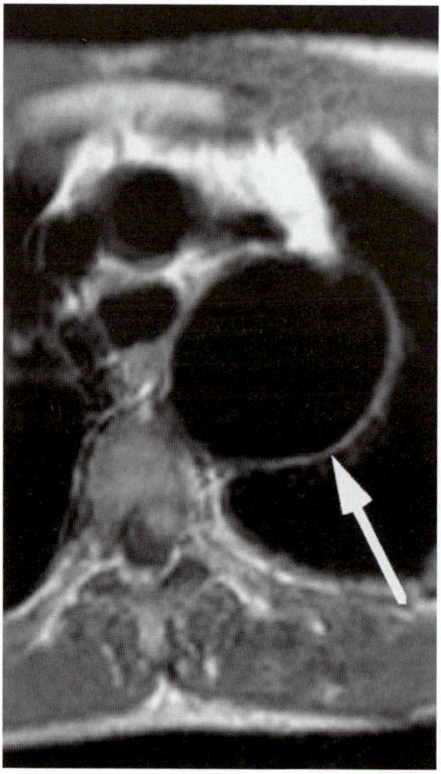

Fig. 3.**9** Transverse spin-echo image in a patient who underwent coarctation repair. A huge false aneurysm is demonstrated (arrow) at the site of repair.

MR imaging was shown to be particularly useful in the non-invasive follow-up of patients after surgical repair (Fig. 3.**8**). Recoarctation, residual stenosis, persistence of aortic arch hypoplasia, postoperative hematoma and false aneurysm at the site of repair can be easily detected and evaluated using MRI techniques [23, 24] (Fig. 3.**9**).

In most cases today, echocardiography and MRI are usually sufficient for the assessment and planning of therapeutic interventions in patients with aortic coarctations.

3.2 Aortic Arch Anomalies

MRI is at present considered as the procedure of choice, superior to echocardiography for identifying aortic arch anomalies because it has the potential to image the vascular abnormalities in multiple planes with a large field of view. MRI allows one to directly image the relationship of vascular structures with the airways and esophagus as well as the degree of tracheal or bronchial compression [25,26,27]. Spin-echo imaging in transverse and coronal planes is usually performed first followed by a 3D gadolinium-enhanced angiographic sequence in the sagittal plane. Source images can be subse-

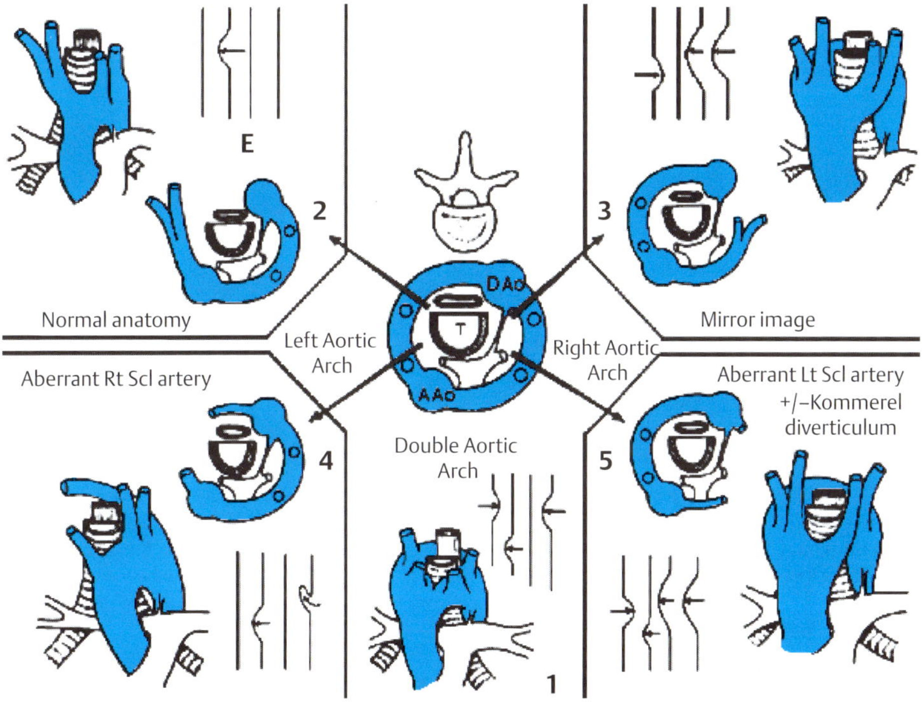

Fig. 3.**10** Edward's hypothetical double aortic arch schema. Compression of the esophagus (E) in AP and lateral projections is indicated in the angle of each diagram. Double aortic arch is due to the persistence of right and left fourth arches both connecting with ascending (AAo) and descending aorta (DAo) (1). Arrows represent the different locations where regression occurs on these both arches leading to normal or abnormal anatomy. In 2, regression occurs behind the right subclavian artery leading to normal anatomy with left aortic arch. 3 represents the mirror image with right aortic arch. In 4, the regression occurs between right carotid and right subclavian arteries leading to aberrant right subclavian artery, originating from the DAo. In 5, the regression occurs between left carotid and left subclavian arteries leading to aberrant left subclavian artery, originating from the DAo and right aortic arch.

quently reconstructed by MIP, surface or volume rendering and MPR techniques in any desirable plane, depending upon the abnormality encountered. The MPR technique can be applied as well on spin-echo images to demonstrate the anomaly of the aortic arch and its relationship with the airways and esophagus (see Fig. 3.**12**).

Double aortic arch is due to the persistence of right and left fourth branchial arches and dorsal aortic roots (Fig. 3.**10**). In double aortic arch, both arches arise from the ascending aorta, pass on both sides of the trachea and the esophagus to join posteriorly and form the descending aorta. Separate common carotid and subclavian arteries arise from each arch. The right arch is usually larger and the left may be atretic or hypoplastic. The upper descending aorta is often right-sided but may occasionally lie to the left of the spine. With the ascending aorta, these arches form a vascular ring

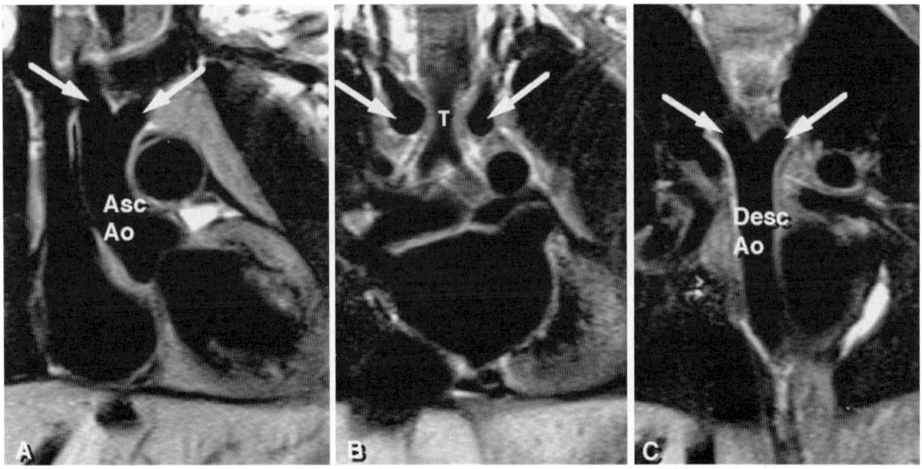

Fig. 3.**11** Coronal spin-echo images (**A** – **C**) of a double aortic arch. Both arches (arrows) arise from the ascending aorta (Asc Ao), pass on both sides of the trachea (T) and the esophagus to join posteriorly and form the descending aorta (Desc Ao). The right arch is larger than the left as usual. With the ascending aorta, these arches form a vascular ring that compresses trachea and esophagus.

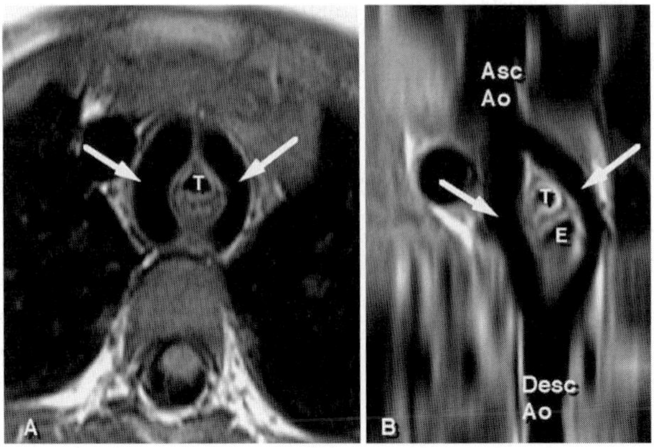

Fig. 3.**12** Transverse spin-echo image (**A**) and curved multiplanar reconstruction of transverse spin-echo images (**B**) of the entire aorta where the whole vessel has been "flattened" and "extended" in one single plane in a patient with double aortic arch. The entire course of both arches (arrows) as well as the connections with ascending (Asc Ao) and descending (Desc Ao) aorta and the degree of compression of trachea (T) and esophagus (E) are well demonstrated.

that may compress trachea and esophagus and thus be responsible for complaints such as stridor and dysphagia. The ductus arteriosus may be on the left or right or may be bilateral although it is usually left-sided. When it is short, the ductus may pull the pulmonary artery backward and the upper descending aorta forward, increasing the degree of compression on the trachea and the esophagus (Figs. 3.**11** to 3.**13**).

An aberrant left subclavian artery with right aortic arch is the result of interruption of the left fourth aortic arch between the left common carotid (LCCA) and left subclavian (LSCA) arteries in Edwards' hypothetical double aortic arch schema (Fig. 3.**10**).

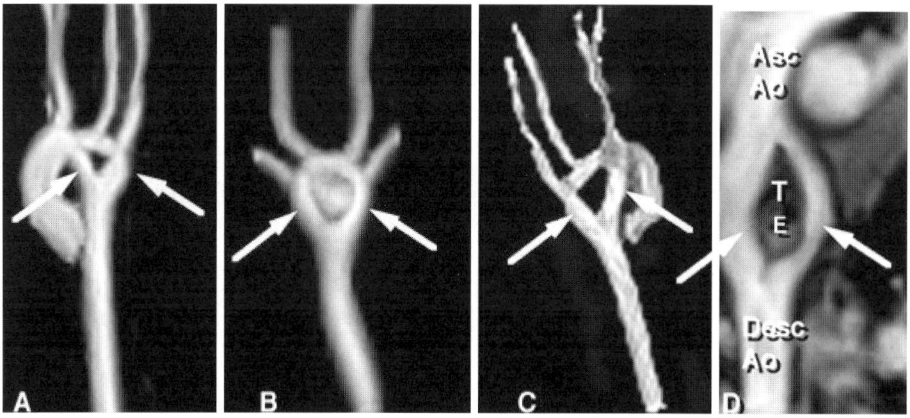

Fig. 3.**13** MIP (**A**, **B**), surface rendering (**C**) and multiplanar reconstruction (MPR) of a 3D gadolinium-enhanced MR angiography (**D**) of the aorta where the whole vessel has been "flattened" and "extended" in one single plane in a patient with double aortic arch. 3D reconstructions help demonstrating the separate arising of common carotid and subclavian arteries from each arch (arrows). The right arch is larger than the left. The degree of compression of trachea (T) and esophagus (E) is also well demonstrated on MPR image.

In this anomaly, the first branch to arise from the aorta is the LCCA, followed by the right common carotid artery (RCCA), the right subclavian artery (RSCA), then the LSCA, as the last branch of the aortic arch. From the aortic arch positioned on the right it courses posterior to the esophagus to reach the left arm. Posterior esophageal compression may occur and be responsible for dysphagia. The descending aorta may lie on either side of the spine but is more often right-sided. The ductus arteriosus or ligamentum arteriosum is more commonly left-sided. The remnant of the left dorsal aortic root may appear as a diverticulum (Kommerell diverticulum) at the origin of the LSCA (Fig. 3.**14**). The ligamentum arteriosum extends from the pulmonary artery to the diverticulum. A symptomatic vascular ring created by the aberrant LSCA consists of the ascending aorta and pulmonary artery in front of the trachea, the aortic arch on the right, the ligamentum arteriosum on the left and the aberrant LSCA with the diverticulum behind the esophagus. The proximal portion of the aberrant LSCA may be stenotic or even atretic.

An aberrant right subclavian artery with left aortic arch is the result of interruption of the right fourth aortic arch between the RCCA and RSCA in Edwards' hypothetical double aortic arch schema (Fig. 3.**10**). Although most patients with this anomaly are asymptomatic, esophageal compression may occur and be responsible for dysphagia ("dysphagia lusoria"). The RSCA is the last branch of the aortic arch and courses posterior to the esophagus to reach the right arm (Fig. 3.**15**). The remnant of this right dorsal aortic root may appear as a diverticulum at the origin of the RSCA and may evolve into aneurysm in the elderly with possible rupture.

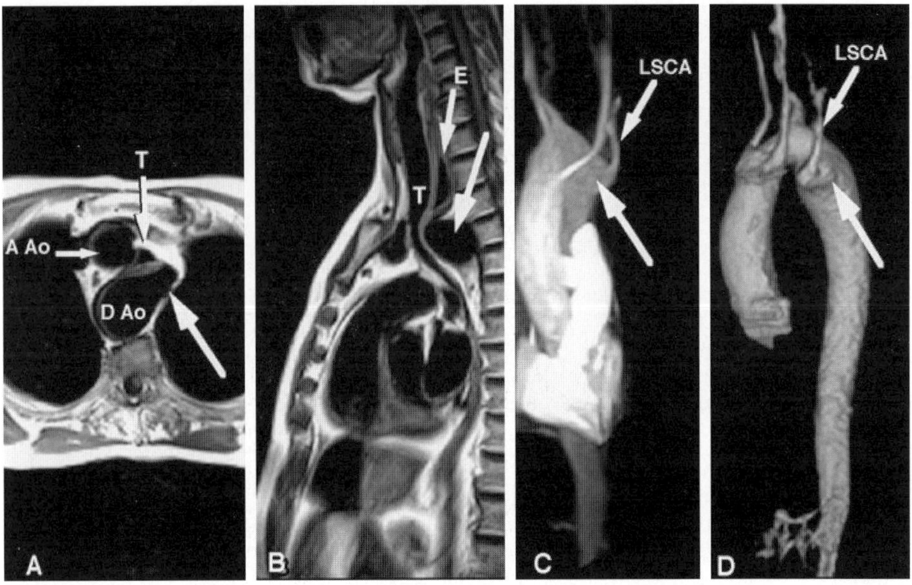

Fig. 3.**14** Patient with aberrant left subclavian artery (LSCA) with right aortic arch and Kommerell diverticulum at the origin of the LSCA. The diverticulum (arrows) compressing the trachea (T) and esophagus (E) is shown on spin-echo images (**A**, **B**) as well as on MIP (**C**) and volume rendering (**D**) reconstructions of a 3D breath-hold gadolinium-enhanced MR angiography.

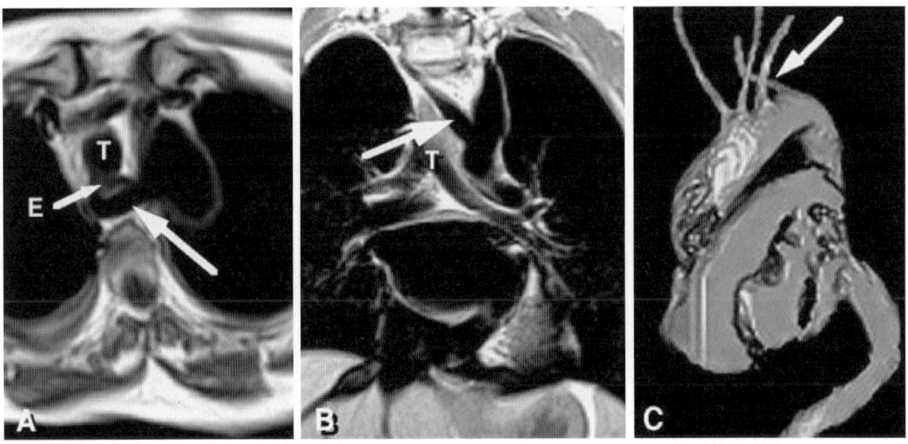

Fig. 3.**15** Left aortic arch with aberrant right subclavian artery (arrows). The abnormal course of the vessel, posterior to the trachea (T) and the esophagus (E) is well shown on transverse (**A**) and coronal (**B**) spin-echo images. Surface rendering of a contrast-enhanced MR angiography (**C**) helps to identify the aberrant artery as the fourth vessel arising from the beginning of the descending aorta.

3.3 Interrupted Aortic Arch

Interruption of the aortic arch is characterized by complete discontinuity (absence of any structural connection) between the ascending and descending aorta. It is a rare anomaly accounting for about 1 percent of congenital heart diseases. It must be distinguished from severe coarctation and aortic atresia in which an imperforate fibrous chord maintains continuity between the aortic segments. The descending aorta in congenital interruption is supplied by a patent ductus arteriosus and by collateral flow from systemic arteries. Aortic arch interruption is classified by the site of interruption relative to the brachiocephalic arteries [28] (Fig. 3.**16**).

- Type A: Discontinuity of the aortic arch distal to the left subclavian artery (44%).
- Type B: Discontinuity between the left subclavian and the left common carotid artery (52%).
- Type C: Interruption between the left common carotid and the innominate artery (4%).

Subgroups: –1 when the right subclavian artery arises normally from the innominate artery; –2 when the right subclavian artery arises anomalously from the distal aortic segment. Associated anomalies are: ventricular septal defect, usually malalignment type with pulmonary hypertension, subaortic stenosis, transposition of the great vessels, bicuspid aortic valve, truncus arteriosus, aortic-pulmonary window, single ventricle and double outlet right ventricle.

MRI can demonstrate the site and the length of the interrupted segment as a high signal intensity tissue at the site of interruption on spin-echo images in the sagittal oblique plane. The malformation may be confirmed by a gadolinium-enhanced 3D MR angiography [29] (Fig. 3.**17**).

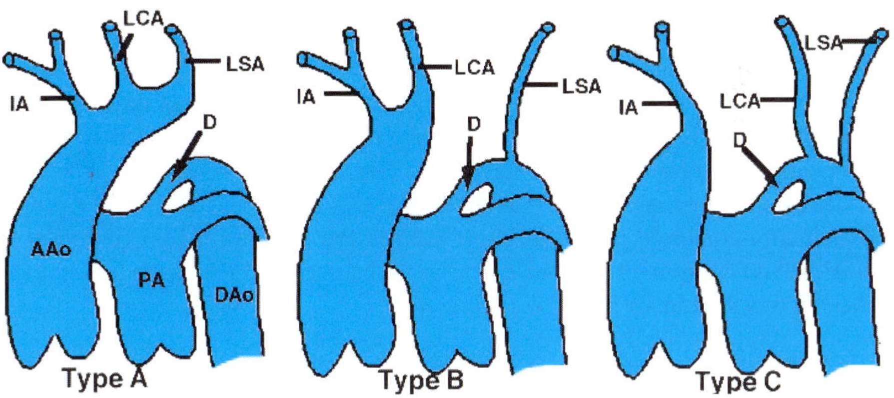

Fig. 3.**16** Scheme of the different types of interrupted aortic arch.
IA = Innominate artery, LCA = left carotid artery, LSA = left subclavian artery, D = ductus arteriosus, AAo = ascending aorta, DAo = descending aorta, PA = pulmonary artery.

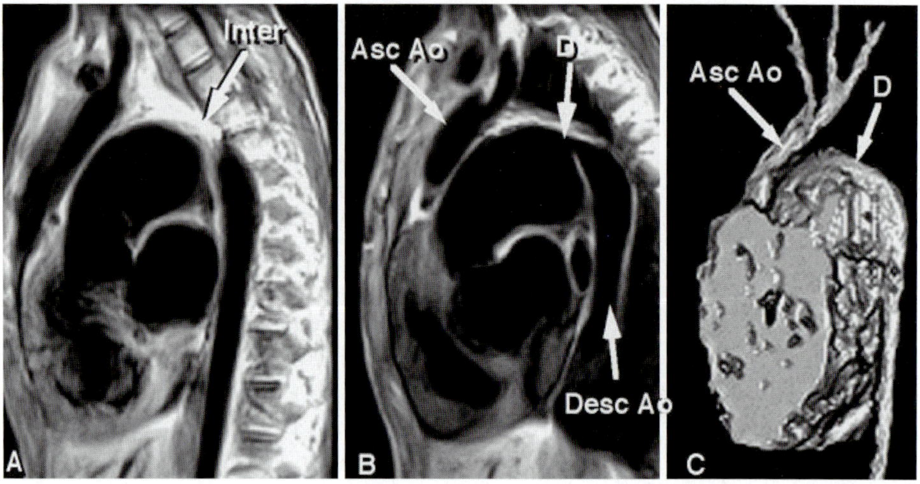

Fig. 3.**17** Oblique sagittal spin-echo images (**A**, **B**) and surface rendering of a 3D breath-hold gadolinium-enhanced MR angiography (**C**) in a patient with type A interrupted aortic arch. The interrupted segment appears as a high signal intensity tissue (Inter) between the ascending (Asc Ao) and descending (Desc Ao) aorta. The flow in descending aorta is supplied by a large patent ductus arteriosus (D).

3.4 Cervical Aortic Arch

Cervical aortic arch is characterized by elongation of the aorta with the apex of the arch in a cervical position. It may be right- or left-sided, although it is more frequently on the right. Persistence of the third aortic arch rather than the fourth is the embryologic explanation the most frequently postulated. A vascular ring may exist depending on the arrangement of brachiocephalic arteries and the position of the ductus arteriosus. The descending aorta may be ipsilateral or contralateral. Associated brachiocephalic artery anomalies are frequent depending on the side of the descending aorta. When there is a contralateral descending aorta, the left subclavian artery may be aberrant, arising from the descending aorta (Fig. 3.**18**). A kinking of the arch in the isthmic region can be encountered as well.

Gadolinium-enhanced breath-hold 3D MRA is the best techniques to detect the anomaly demonstrating the anomalous arch in the neck and the associated brachiocephalic artery anomalies [30].

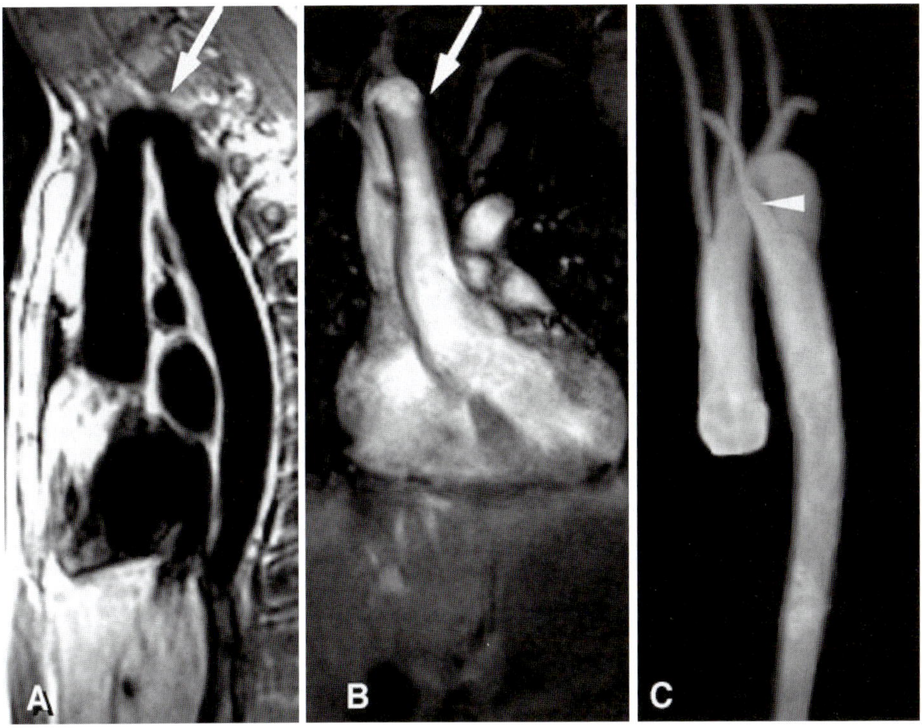

Fig. 3.**18** Oblique sagittal spin-echo (**A**), coronal cine-GE (**B**) images and maximum intensity projection of a 3D breath-hold gadolinium-enhanced MR angiography (**C**) in a patient with a cervical aortic arch (arrows). The descending aorta is right-sided and the left subclavian artery is aberrant, arising from the descending aorta (arrow-head).

3.5 Aortic Aneurysms

Aortic aneurysms are classified into two morphologic types: fusiform which encompasses the circumference of the vessel with a spindle shape and saccular where a pouch protrudes from the aortic wall with a narrow neck. True aneurysms are defined as localized enlargements in which all layers of the aortic wall are present whereas false aneurysms (pseudoaneurysms) are localized enlargements of the vessel in which the wall consists of the adventitia only or fibrous tissue.

Aneurysms of the ascending aorta are located from aortic annulus to the origin of the innominate artery. They can be associated with dilatation of the sinuses of Valsalva and aortic annulus (annulo-aortic ectasia) responsible for aortic valve insufficiency. They can be isolated or associated with Marfan syndrome where the ascending aorta may undergo progressive dilatation leading to severe regurgitation or may be complicated by type A aortic dissection. Other etiologies include congenital, aortitis (due to syphilis or other causes), arteriosclerosis, post-traumatic, poststenotic dilatation (jet lesion) from aortic stenosis and infection. MRI and particularly MR angiogra-

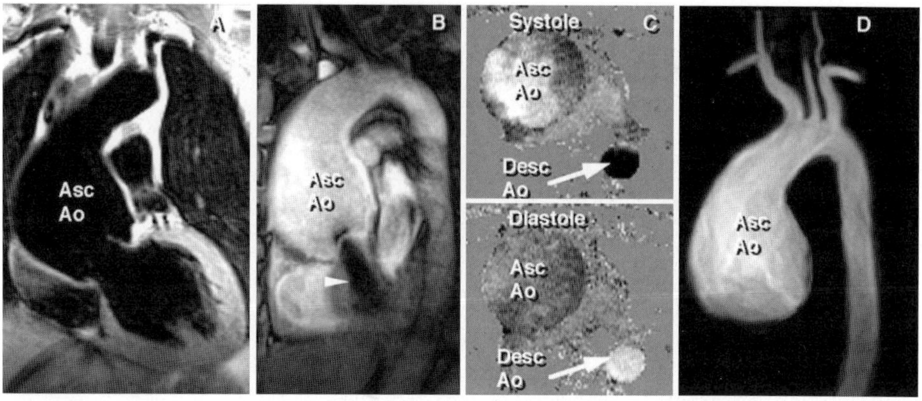

Fig. 3.**19** Coronal spin-echo (**A**), oblique sagittal cine-GE (**B**), transverse velocity-encoded cine (VEC) (**C**) and MIP (**D**) images of a patient with a Marfan syndrome and aneurysm of the ascending aorta (Asc Ao). The dilatation includes aortic annulus and sinus of Valsalva and is responsible for aortic regurgitation, well demonstrated as a long flow void (arrow-head) on diastolic cine-GE image. VEC images show an antegrade flow (bright signal intensity) in the Asc Ao in systole and a retrograde flow (dark signal intensity) in diastole. The signal intensity in the descending aorta (Desc Ao) is opposite to that of the Asc Ao. It allowed the calculation of a regurgitant fraction of 70% indicating a severe aortic regurgitation (see Chapter 5 and fourth section of the CD ROM).

phy (MRA) play an important role in monitoring non-invasively the degree of enlargement of the ascending aorta [31,32,33]. With the help of associated gated-cine and velocity-encoded sequences, the method allows one to assess quantitatively the degree of associated valvular regurgitation (Fig. 3.**19**).

Aortic arch aneurysms may be fusiform involving the entire aortic arch or saccular developing either laterally or inferiorly in the aortopulmonary window. Most frequent etiologies are arteriosclerosis, syphilis and post-traumatic (pseudoaneurysms) usually located distal to the left subclavian artery. MRI and particularly MR angiography provide an accurate method for the detection, outer diameter measurement and characterization of these aneurysms and their extension and location in relation to the brachiocephalic vessels. MR images allow one to detect a mural thrombus as well (Fig. 3.**20**). This thrombus appears as an intermediate signal intensity structure within the aneurysm on spin-echo images. Areas of high signal intensity within the thrombus may indicate instability of the aneurysm [33]. Cine-GE images permit the differentiation between the thrombus and associated slow flow within the aneurysm, which can also produce an intraluminal signal on depicting a mural filling defect. 3D contrast MRA is the best technique to provide a comprehensive overview of the aneurysm due to the cross-sectional information provided by source images and the different reconstruction techniques. The thrombosed part of the aneurysm will be well depicted on source images whereas it will be completely obscured on an MIP reconstruction that displays only the circulating lumina [22]. In some cases, differentiation between true and false aneurysms is possible. In general, a large connection

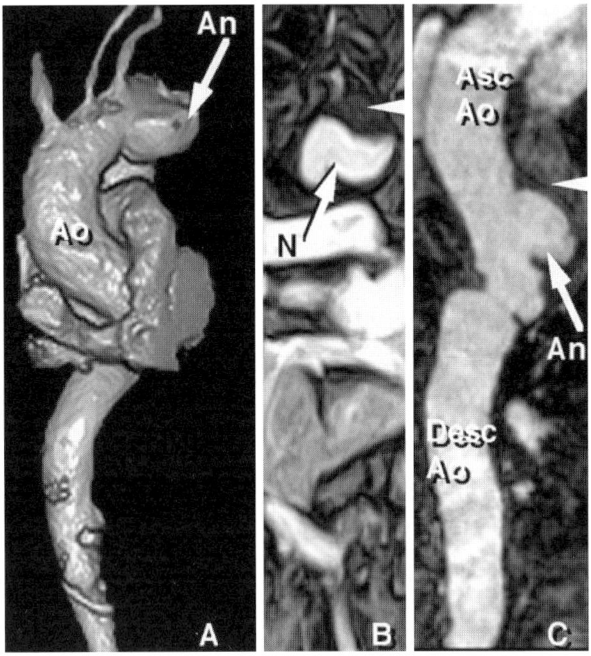

Fig. 3.**20** Contrast-enhanced MR angiography in a patient with an aneurysm (An) of the aortic arch. Surface rendering image (**A**) shows the relationship of the aneurysm with the brachiocephalic vessels (situated at the level of left subclavian artery) but the neck and the thrombus are not visible. Both coronal (**B**) and curved elongated arch (**C**) MPR images display the saccular morphology of the aneurysm as well as the neck (N) and intra-aneurysmal thrombus (arrow-heads).

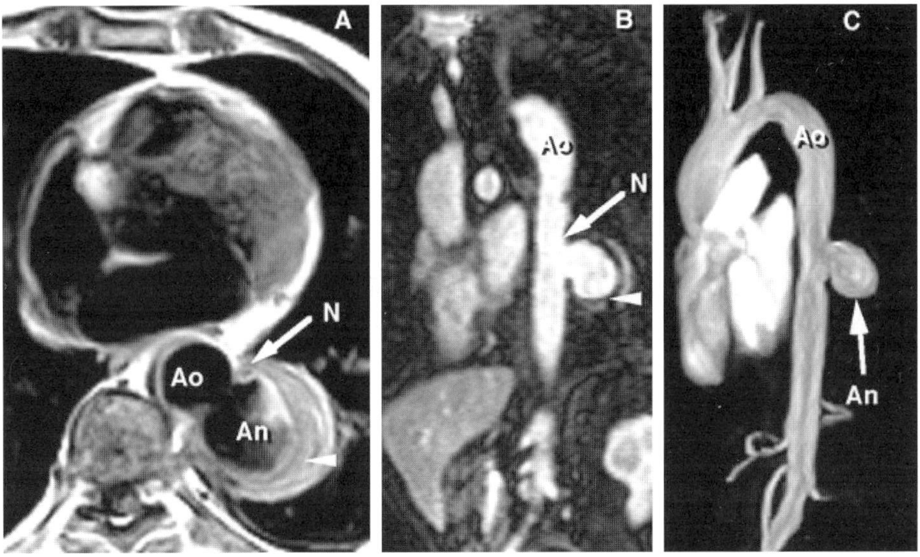

Fig. 3.**21** Transverse spin-echo (**A**) and contrast-enhanced MR angiography (**B**, **C**) images in a patient with a saccular aneurysm (An) of the descending aorta. Spin-echo images show the aneurysm (An) with a narrow neck (N). Peripheral medium signal intensity (arrow-head) corresponds to thrombus and slow blood flow within the An. Source images of MR angiography (**B**) and MIP reconstruction (**C**) confirm the An with its narrow neck. Mural thrombus is only shown on source images surrounded by enhanced aneurysmal wall (arrow-head).

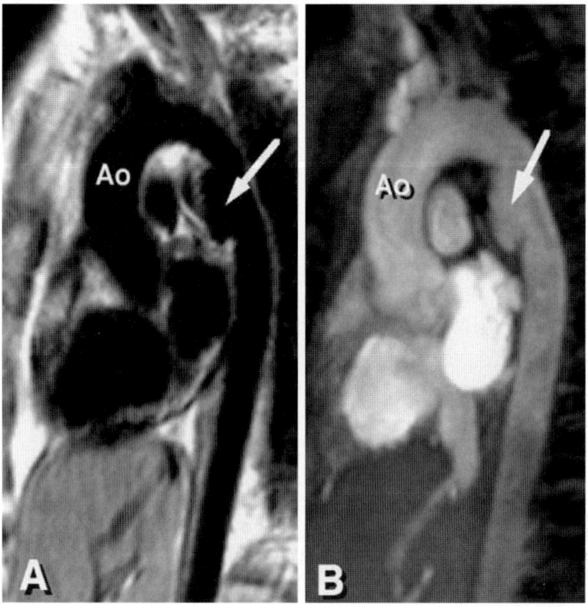

Fig. 3.**22** Oblique sagittal spin-echo (**A**) and cine-MIP (**B**) images of a patient with a post-traumatic pseudoaneurysm of the aorta. The focal enlargement of the isthmus with irregularities of the aortic wall (arrows) is well shown.

with the aortic lumen indicates that it is a true aneurysm whereas a narrow neck with saccular expansion is more often a sign of a pseudoaneurysm. One limitation of MRI is its inability to demonstrate calcifications.

Aneurysms of the descending aorta are usually due to arteriosclerosis (fusiform; true aneurysms) or infection (saccular; pseudoaneurysms). MRA is an accurate method for the detection, measurement, survey and planning for surgery or stent-graft treatment of these aneurysms [34] (Fig. 3.**21**).

Post-traumatic pseudoaneurysms are almost all caused by non-penetrating trauma, most often due to rapid deceleration in an automobile accident. 20% of the patients survive the initial event due to formation of a periaortic hematoma and false aneurysm contained by the adventitia and surrounding tissues.

Most post-traumatic pseudoaneurysms occur near the aortic isthmus, just distal to the insertion of ligamentum arteriosum at the junction of mobile and fixed aorta.

MRI demonstrates the false aneurysm, with enlargement and circumferential deformity of the aortic wall at the level of the isthmus [33]. Other signs are more subtle: initial descending aorta is larger in caliber than ascending aorta, indicating aneurysm, changes in aortic contours such as irregularities of the aortic wall, intimal tear may be observed. Gated cine angiography as well as gadolinium-enhanced breath-hold 3D MRA are the best techniques to demonstrate the false aneurysm (Fig. 3.**22**).

3.6 Aortic Dissections

Diagnosis of acute aortic dissection relies so far on transesophageal echocardiography and multislice spiral CT. MRI plays an important role as a non-invasive technique in the follow-up of Stanford type B dissection treated medically as well as Stanford type A aortic dissection. The latter is usually treated immediately by ascending aorta replacement either by Dacron prosthesis with aortic valve conservation and repair of proximal and distal portions of dissections with biological glue or Bentall intervention [33, 34, 35].

MRA, which is very sensitive to flow alterations in the true and false lumens, allows detection of unknown complications.

MRI images may demonstrate: ascending aorta aneurysm proximal to the prosthesis without recurrent dissection but with aortic regurgitation or recurrent dissection proximal to the prosthesis with two patent lumens with or without aortic regurgitation. A pseudoaneurysm proximal, at the level or distal to the prosthesis at suture lines may be detected as well. Aneurysms of isthmic and descending aortic false lumen can be monitored. MRI also allows the detection of several entry points of the dissection in order to plan a stent-graft placement, shows the persistence or recurrence of dissection distal to the prosthesis with patency of true and false channels, partial or complete thrombosis of the false lumen distal to the prosthesis and the degree of compression of the true lumen by the false channel (Figs. 3.**23** to 3.**25**).

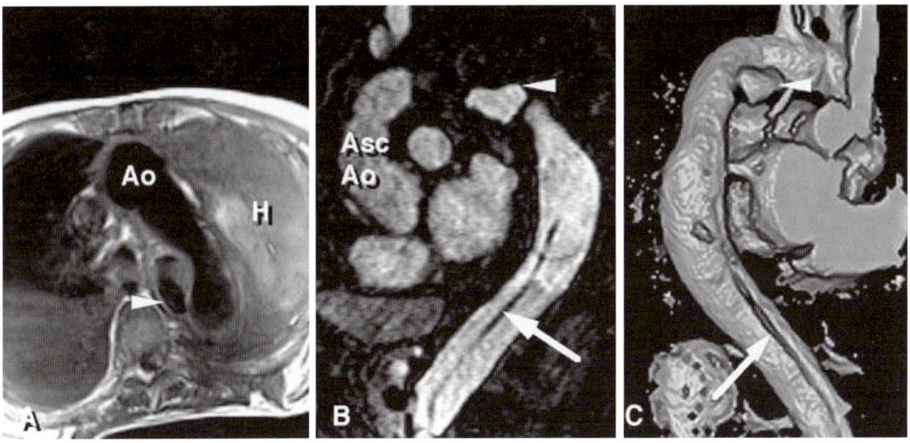

Fig. 3.**23** Type A aortic dissection s/p ascending aorta (Asc Ao) and aortic arch replacement by a Dacron graft. Spin-echo image (**A**) demonstrates an extensive hemothorax (H) and a pseudoaneurysm (PSA) (arrow-head) at sutures lines of aortic arch prosthesis. 3D MRA source images (**B**) and surface rendering images (**C**) show the PSA (arrow-head) originating from the fifth intercostal artery and persisting intimal flap in descending aorta (arrow).

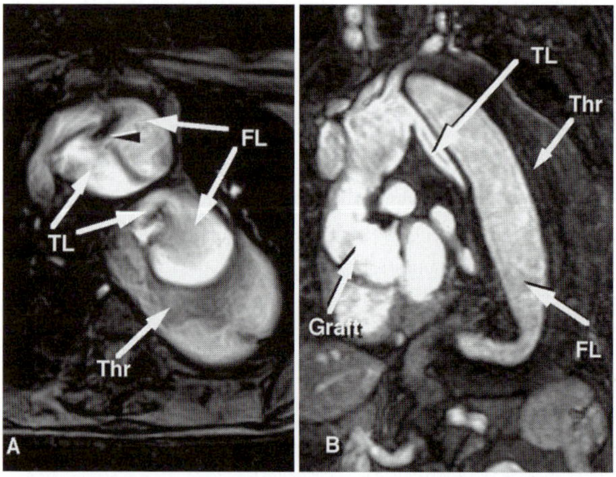

Fig. 3.**24** Type A aortic dissection s/p ascending aorta replacement by a Dacron graft. Cine-GE images (**A**) show a residual entry point (arrow-head) in ascending aorta distal to the graft. In descending aorta, the false lumen (FL) is aneurysmal and there is extensive mural thrombus (Thr). 3D MRA source images (**B**) better demonstrate the aneurysmal and thrombosed FL, compressing the true lumen (TL) and absence of anomaly at the level of the graft.

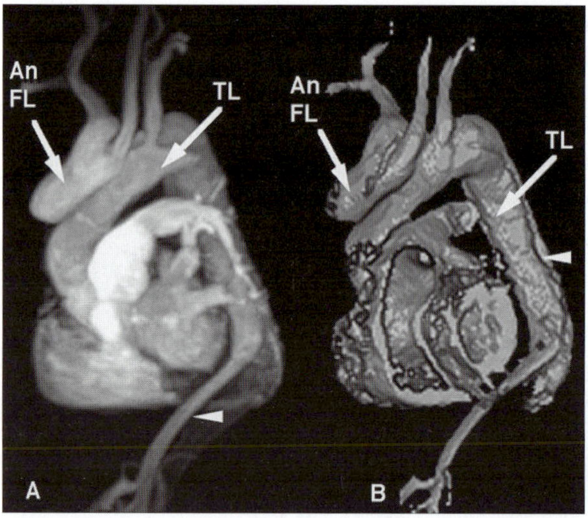

Fig. 3.**25** Type A aortic dissection s/p ascending aorta replacement by a graft. MIP (**A**) and 3D surface rendering (**B**) images of a contrast-enhanced MRA show innominate and carotid arteries originating from the aneurysmal false lumen (An FL) whereas the left subclavian artery originates from the true lumen (TL). Distally, the intimal flap (arrow-head) is well identified on both reconstruction techniques and the TL is compressed by the FL.

3.7 Aortitis

Arteritis may affect the aorta and its branches. The main cause is Takayasu's disease. Aortitis can be encountered as well in giant cell arteritis, ankylosing spondylitis, psoriasis, ulcerative colitis, Behçet's disease, relapsing polychondritis and Reiter's syndrome. MRI findings consist of aortic wall thickening isolated or associated with either constriction or aneurysmal dilatation. Frequently, a dilated segment is interposed between two narrowed ones [33].

In Takayasu's aortitis an inflammatory process of unknown etiology affects the aorta and its major branches. Pulmonary arteries may be affected as well. Intimal proliferation associated with degeneration of the elastic fibers of the media is the

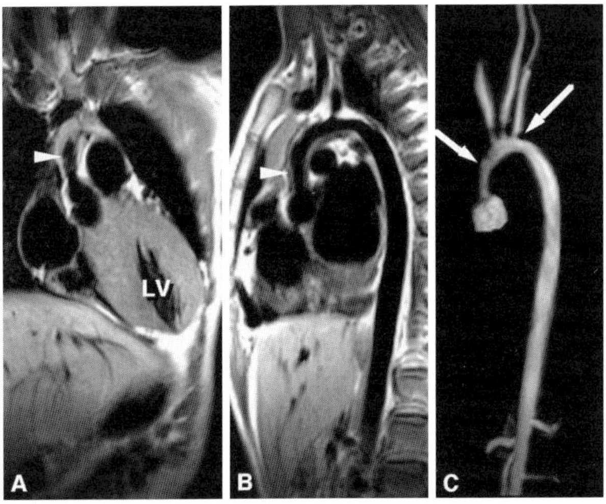

Fig. 3.**26** Coronal (**A**), oblique sagittal (**B**) spin-echo and 3D MRA MIP (**C**) images of a young boy with Takayasu's disease. Spin-echo images show a severe stenosis of ascending aorta associated with wall thickening (arrow-head) and left ventricle hypertrophy. MIP reconstruction demonstrates the involvement of all the brachiocephalic vessels by the arteritis with severe stenosis (arrows).

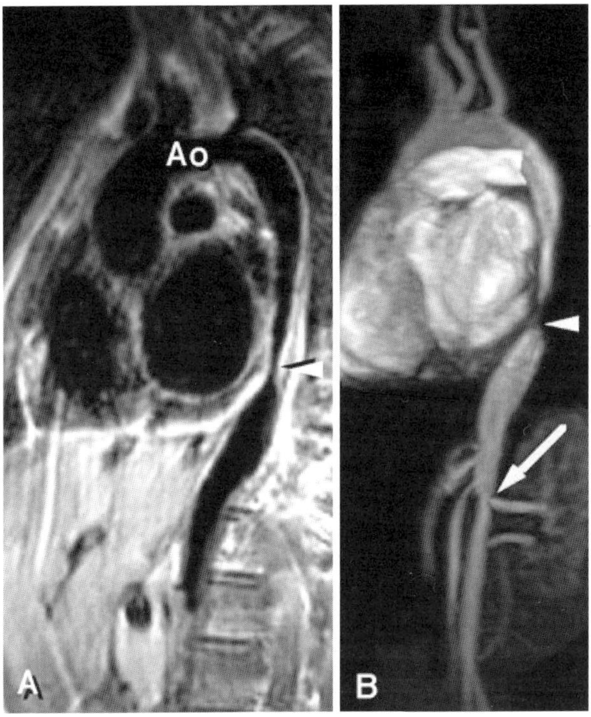

Fig. 3.**27** Oblique sagittal spin-echo (**A**) and 3D MRA MIP (**B**) images of a patient with Takayasu's disease involving descending and abdominal aorta. Spin-echo images show a severe stenosis of descending aorta associated with wall thickening (arrow-head). MIP images overestimate the degree of stenosis of the descending aorta and show involvement of abdominal aorta as well (arrow).

initial lesion. The disease consists of one or a combination of the following signs: mural thickening of the ascending aorta, aortic arch and their branches with stenosis or occlusion of arch vessels which is the most common variety (Fig. 3.**26**). Involvement of descending aorta or abdominal aorta and its branches with pseudocoarctation is less common (Fig. 3.**27**).

3.8 Aortic Thrombus

In cases of ischemia of the upper extremities or peripheral embolization, echocardiography is the first screening modality in order to detect the source of the embolus. The most frequent sites of thrombus are the left ventricle in cases of cardiomyopathies or recent infarction or the left atrium in cases of mitral disease and/or atrial fibrillation. Less frequently, the source of embolization may be the aorta. MRI, with its large field of view, its multiplanar capability and its sensibility to flow abnormalities is the procedure of choice to demonstrate thrombi in the aorta [36].

Gated cine angiography and gadolinium-enhanced breath-hold 3D MRA are the best techniques to detect the thrombus, appearing as low signal intensity filling defect in the vessel on cine-GE and the source images of MRA. On maximum-intensity projection (MIP) images, the thrombus may be partially or completely obscured by the reconstruction technique (Fig. 3.**28**).

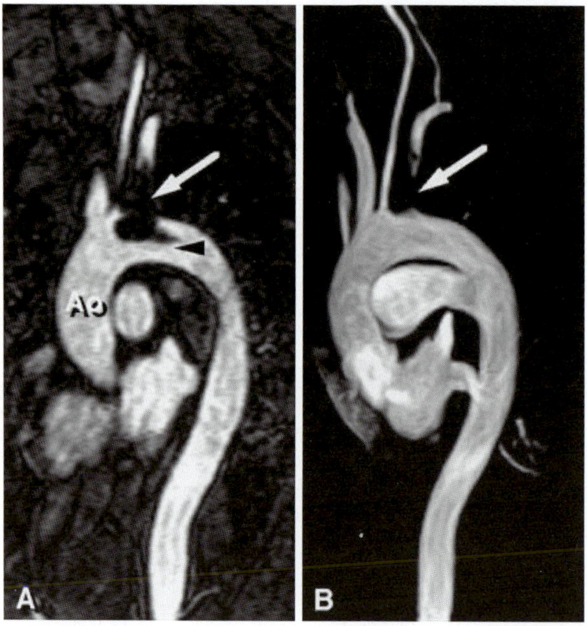

Fig. 3.**28** 3D contrast-enhanced MRA of a patient with aortic thrombus (**A**). A low signal intensity in the aortic arch (arrow-head) and the origin of left subclavian artery (arrow) is well demonstrated on source images corresponding to the thrombus. On MIP images (**B**) the filling defect in the aortic arch is obscured by the reconstruction technique. Only the left subclavian artery obstruction is detected (arrow).

3.9 References

1. Harnell GG, Finn JP, Zenni M, et al. MR imaging of the thoracic aorta: comparison of spin-echo, angiographic and breath-hold techniques. Radiology 1994; 191: 697–704.
2. Higgins CB. The vascular system. Magnetic resonance imaging of the body. Raven Press, New York, 1992, pp 629–667.
3. Didier D, Ratib O, Beghetti M, et al. Morphologic and functional evaluation of congenital heart disease by magnetic resonance imaging. J Magn Reson Imaging 1999; 10: 639–655.
4. Higgins CB, Silvermann NH, Kersting-Sommerhoff BA, Schmid TK. Congenital heart disease. Echocardiography and Magnetic Resonance Imaging. Raven Press, New York, 1990.
5. Link KM, Lesko NM. The role of MR imaging in the evaluation of acquired diseases of the thoracic aorta. AJR 1992; 158: 1115–1125.
6. Nayler GL, Firmin DN, Longmore DB. Blood flow imaging by cine magnetic resonance. J Comput Assist Tomography 1987; 10: 715–722.
7. Wexler L, Higgins CB. The use of magnetic resonance imaging in adult congenital heart disease. Am J Card Imaging 1995; 9: 15–28.
8. Ho VB, Prince MR. Thoracic MR aortography: Imaging techniques and strategies. RadioGraphics 1998; 18: 287–309.
9. Prince MR, Narasimham DL, Jacoby WT, et al. Three-dimensional gadolinium-enhanced MR angiography of the thoracic aorta. AJR 1996; 166: 1387–1397.
10. Krinsky GA, Rofsky NM, Flyer M, et al. Thoracic aorta: comparison of gadolinium-enhanced three-dimensional MR angiography and conventional MR imaging. Radiology 1997; 202: 183–193.
11. Prince MR. Contrast-enhanced MR angiography: Theory and optimization. MRI Clin North Am 1998; 6: 257–267.
12. Didier D, Higgins CB, Fisher MR, et al. Gated magnetic resonance imaging in congenital heart disease: experience in initial 72 patients. Radiology 1986; 158: 227–235.
13. Fletcher BD, Jacobstein MD. MRI of congenital abnormalities of the great arteries. AJR 1986; 146: 941–948.
14. Amparo EG, Higgins CB, Schafton EG. Demonstration of coarctation of the aorta by magnetic resonance imaging. AJR 1984; 143: 1192–1194.
15. Von Shulthess GK, Higashino SM, Higgins SS, Didier D, Fisher MR, Higgins CB. Coarctation of the aorta : MR imaging. Radiology 1986; 158: 469–474.
16. Didier D, Ratib O, Friedli B, et al. Cine gradient-echo MR imaging in the evaluation of cardiovascular diseases. RadioGraphics 1993; 13: 561–573.
17. Rebergen SA, Niezen RA, Helbing WA, van der Wall EE, de Roos A, Cine gradient echo MR imaging and MR velocity mapping in the evaluation of congenital heart disease. RadioGraphics 1996; 16: 467–481.
18. Bogren HG, Buonocore MH: Blood flow measurements in the aorta and major arteries with MR velocity mapping. JMRI 1994; 4: 119–130.

19. Firmin D, Underwood R. Magnetic resonance flow imaging. In: Magnetic Resonance of the cardiovascular system. Underwood R, Firmin D (eds), Blackwell Scientific Publications, Oxford, 1991.
20. Mohiaddin RH, Pennell DJ. MR blood flow measurement. Clinical application in the heart and circulation. Cardiol Clin 1998; 16: 161–187.
21. Szolar DH, Sakuma H, Higgins CB. Cardiovascular applications of magnetic resonance flow and velocity measurements. JMRI 1996; 1: 78–89.
22. Prince MR, Grist TM, Debatin JF. 3D contrast MR angiography. Springer Verlag, Berlin, 1997.
23. Muhler EG, Neuerburg JM,, Ruben A, et al. Evaluation of aortic coarctation after surgical repair: role of magnetic resonance imaging and Doppler ultrasound. Br Heart J 1993; 70: 285–290.
24. Bogaert J, Kuzo R, Dymarkowski S, et al. Follow-up of patients with previous treatment for coarctation of the thoracic aorta: comparison between contrast-enhanced MR angiography and fast spin-echo imaging. Eur Radiol 2000; 10: 1847–1854.
25. Bisset GS, Strife GL, Kirks DR, Bailey WW. Vascular rings – MR imaging. AJR 1987; 149: 251–256.
26. Gomes AS, Lois JF, George B, et al. Congenital anomalies of the aortic arch: MR imaging. Radiology 1987; 165: 691–695.
27. Kersting-Sommerhoff BA, Sechtem UP, Fisher MR, Higgins CB. MR imaging of congenital anomalies of the aortic arch. AJR 1987; 149: 9–13.
28. Neye-Bock S, Fellows KE. Aortic arch interruption in infancy: Radio- and angiographic features. AJR 1980; 135: 1005–1010.
29. Roche KJ, Krinsky G, Lee VS, et al. Interrupted aortic arch: diagnosis with gadolinium-enhanced 3D MRA. J Comput Assist Tomogr 1999; 23: 197–202.
30. Soler R, Rodriguez E, Requejo I, et al. Magnetic resonance imaging of congenital abnormalities of the thoracic aorta. Eur Radiol 1998; 8: 540–546.
31. Soulen RL, Fishman EK, Pyeritz RE, et al. Marfan syndrome: evaluation with MR imaging versus CT. Radiology 1987; 165: 697–701.
32. Dinsmore RE, Liberthson RR, Wismer GL, et al. Magnetic resonance imaging of thoracic aortic aneurysms: comparison of other imaging methods. AJR 1986; 147: 253–256.
33. Fattori R, Nienaber CA. MRI of acute and chronic aortic pathology: pre-operative and postoperative evaluation. J Magn Reson Imaging 1999; 10: 741–750.
34. Hartnell GG. Imaging of aortic aneurysms and dissection: CT and MRI. J Thorac Imaging 2001; 16: 35–46.
35. Schmidt M, Theissen P, Klempt G et al. Long term follow-up of 82 patients with chronic disease of the thoracic aorta using spin-echo and cine gradient magnetic resonance imaging. Magn Reson Imaging 2000; 18: 795–806.
36. Seelos KC, Funari M, Higgins CB. Detection of aortic arch thrombus using MR imaging. J Comput Assist Tomog 1991; 15: 244–247.

4 Cardiac Masses

Cardiac tumors are relatively rare but represent a clinically significant subtype of cardiac-related diseases that benefit from MR imaging techniques. Even benign tumors that are readily treatable and curable can result in significant morbidity if not detected appropriately. This chapter also covers a broader range of related diseases under the generic title of "cardiac masses" encompassing non-tumoral masses such as thrombi, cysts and valvular vegetations. With the ability of MRI to accurately localize and differentiate abnormal soft tissue structures as well as to dynamically evaluate the functional and hemodynamic consequences of anomalous morphological changes, MR imaging has evolved as the imaging modality of choice for the assessment of cardiac and pericardial masses [1,2].

4.1 Classification and Characterization of Cardiac Masses

Cardiac tumors can be divided into primary or secondary tumors. The primary group can be further divided into benign and malignant tumors. A third category will regroup all non-neoplastic conditions and non-tumoral cardiac masses.

4.2 Primary Cardiac Tumors – Benign Tumors

Primary benign cardiac tumors are relatively rare but can cause significant morbidity and mortality. They are usually treatable and can be detected in most cases with echocardiography, but tomographic methods such as CT and MR have emerged as better techniques for more elaborate and accurate assessment of the morphology and extension of these tumors. Both techniques have the advantage of imaging the entire chest and allowing evaluation of the extracardiac extent of the disease. While CT has the capability of detecting calcifications, which is an important variable in the differential diagnosis of cardiac neoplasms, MR imaging has a better soft-tissue contrast than CT and allows much greater flexibility in the selection of imaging planes [3].

4.2.1 Myxoma

Myxomas comprise 50% of primary cardiac tumors and are more common in females. Systemic embolization is one mode of clinical presentation of left atrial myxomas. Emboli can consist of tumor fragments or thrombus from the surface of the tumor. The other modes of presentation are obstruction of blood flow with symptoms of

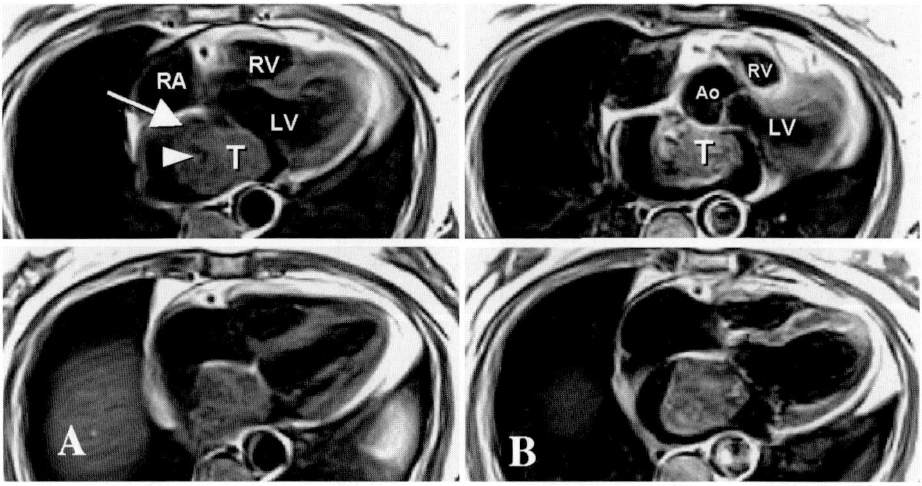

Fig. 4.**1** Left atrial myxoma.
Transverse T1w SE images before (**A**) and after (**B**) gadolinium injection. Tumor (T) is spherical, with a broad attachment to the atrial septum (arrow). It is characterized by an intermediate signal intensity and heterogeneous aspect. Areas of low signal intensity (arrow head) represent partial calcifications. Tumor is enhanced after gadolinium injection.
T = tumor, RA = right atrium, LV = left ventricle, RV = right ventricle, Ao = aorta.

mitral stenosis and systemic constitutional manifestations such as fever, weight loss, anemia and fatigue. Small tumors are often asymptomatic and discovered incidentally. The most frequent localization is the left atrium (left to right ratio of 4:1) and the common site of attachment is the atrial septum near the fossa ovalis. The tumor is usually spherical-shaped, polypoid and may be pedunculated, allowing it to protrude across the mitral valve in diastole, or broad-based. Histologically, the tumor is composed of endothelial-like cells within a myxoid stroma. Areas of hemorrhage are common and hemosiderin is found in varying amounts. Calcifications are rare but may be present.

Echocardiography is the first diagnostic procedure but MRI can play a role in atypical cases [4,5,6]. On SE images, myxomas are characterized by intermediate signal intensity, similar to the myocardium, are homogeneous or heterogeneous due to the presence of areas of low signal intensity (calcifications) or high signal intensity (hemorrhage) (Figs. 4.**1** and 4.**3**). On cine-GE images, the mass appears as a filling defect with low signal intensity compared to the blood (Figs. 4.**2** and 4.**3**). The tumor enhances both on SE and cine GE images with gadolinium which generally excludes the possibility that the mass is a thrombus. The attachment of the mass to the atrial septum, particularly well demonstrated on dynamic images, reinforces the diagnosis of myxoma. The characteristic narrow stalk is the most important distinguishing feature of a myxoma, followed by tumor mobility and distensibility. Tumor location is the other important distinguishing factor. A mass that rises from the interatrial

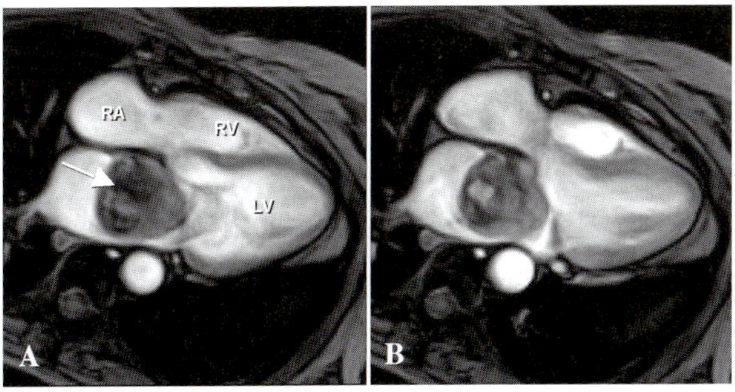

Fig. 4.2 Left atrial myxoma. Transverse cine gradient-echo images obtained in diastole (**A**) and systole (**B**). Note the mobility of the mass protruding through the mitral valve. (see CD ROM for dynamic cine images of this case).
RA = right atrium, LV = left ventricle, RV = right ventricle.

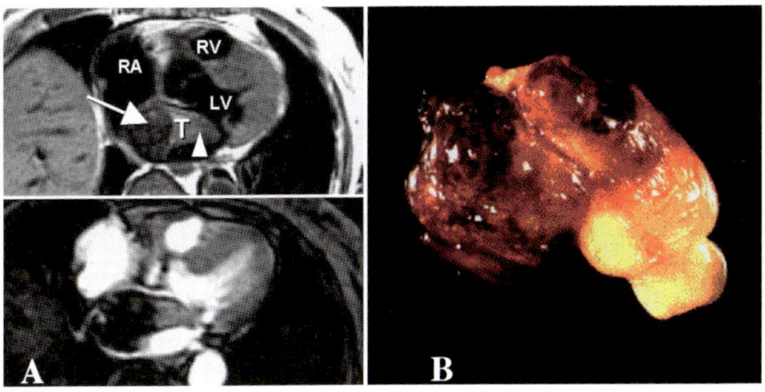

Fig. 4.3 Example of surgically extracted atrial myxoma.
(**A**) MRI images on the left: SE (top image) and cine-GE (bottom image). he tumor shows two components: distal fibrous part (arrow heads) which was protruding in the left ventricle and hemorrhagic basal part (arrow). (**B**) Gross anatomy of the tumor after surgical extraction.
RA = right atrium, LA = left atrium, LV = left ventricle, RV = right ventricle, Ao = aorta.

septum from a narrow base of attachment may be identified as a cardiac myxoma with a high degree of confidence [7].

4.2.2 Lipoma and Lipomatous Atrial Septum

True cardiac lipomas are rare. They can be subendocardic or located within the myocardium responsible for cardiac arrhythmia. The most frequent location is the right atrium [8]. Lipomatous hypertrophy of the atrial septum is more frequent, particularly in obese, elderly patients [9]. Unlike cardiac lipomas, lipomatous hypertrophy of the atrial septum is not encapsulated and is not a true neoplasm (Fig. 4.**4**). It is due to infiltration of the atrial septum by adipose tissue and may be responsible for supraventricular arrhythmia. Usually asymptomatic, lipomatous hypertrophy of the atrial septum is discovered incidentally by echocardiography carried out for other reasons. The mass appears hyperechogenic at ultrasound examination and, of course, is nonspecific. The MRI appearance is characteristic showing, on T1-weighted SE images, a high signal intensity mass within the atrial septum with the same signal intensity as subcutaneous fat. It has the same signal as fat in other sequences such as T2-weighted SE and cine. If a doubt persists, fat-suppression techniques may help in demonstrating

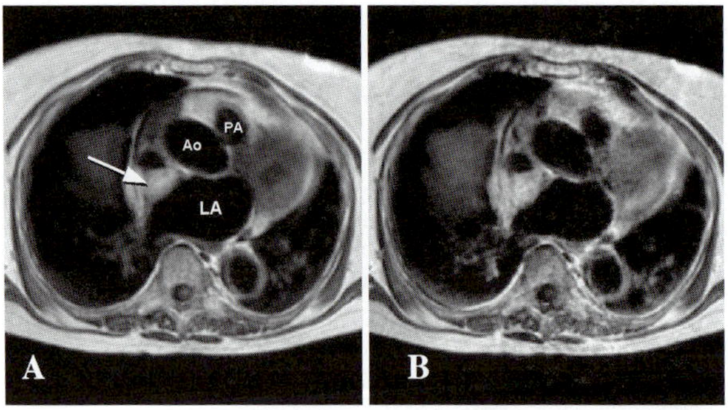

Fig. 4.**4** Lipomatous atrial septum.
Transverse T1w SE images before (**A**) and after (**B**) gadolinium injection. A high signal intensity mass (arrow) with a signal similar to subcutaneous fat is showed in the upper portion of the atrial septum. There is no significant enhancement after gadolinium injection.
LA = left atrium, Ao = aorta, PA = pulmonary artery.

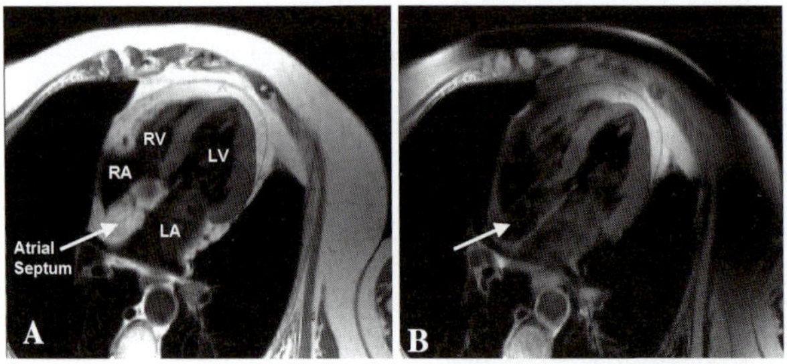

Fig. 4.**5** Lipomatous atrial septum.
Transverse T1w SE images obtained without (**A**) and with (**B**) fat suppression pulse showing that the high signal intensity of fat tissue disappears after fat suppression.
LA = left atrium, RA = right atrium, LV = left ventricle, RV = right ventricle.

reduction of signal in the mass as in subcutaneous fat (Fig. 4.**5**). Like soft-tissue lipomas, cardiac lipomas do not enhance with the administration of contrast material. MRI, with the help of a larger field of view and the multisectional capability is more effective for demonstrating the exact location and the extent as well as the nature of the mass.

4.2.3 Fibroma

Fibroma is a tumor that primarily affects children and in most cases is detected in infants or in utero. At autopsy, fibromas are the second most common benign primary cardiac tumor in children after rhabdomyoma. Cardiac fibromas are often associated with arrhythmias and are the second most common primary cardiac tumor associated with sudden death. About one-third of cardiac fibromas are asymptomatic and may be discovered incidentally. Because of their dense, fibrous nature, the tumors are usually homogeneous and hypointense on T2-weighted MR images and isointense relative to muscle on T1-weighted images. For the same reason, the tumors often demonstrate little or no contrast material enhancement (Fig. 4.**6**). In infants, the primary differential diagnosis for an intramural mass is a rhabdomyoma. If there are multiple masses or signs of tuberous sclerosis, rhabdomyoma can be confidently diagnosed. If the tumor is solitary, ventricular, and calcified, the diagnosis of fibroma can be made from the radiologic findings [11].

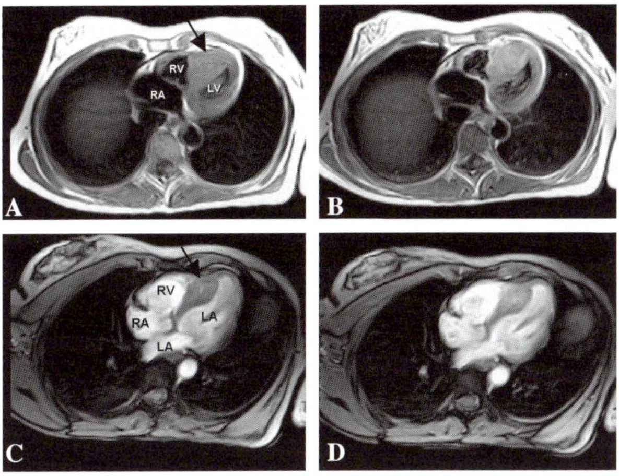

Fig. 4.6 Fibroma of the interventricular septum.
T1w SE images before (**A**) and after (**B**) gadolinium injection and cine gradient-echo (GE) images before (**C**) and after (**D**) gadolinium injection. The tumor shows only moderate increase in signal intensity after Gd injection.
RV = right ventricle, LV = left ventricle, RA = right atrium, LA = left atrium.

4.2.4 Rhabdomyomas

Rhabdomyomas are the most frequent cardiac tumors in infancy and childhood and are frequently associated with tuberous sclerosis [10, 11]. They may be symptomatic usually in the first days or weeks of life by demonstrating cardiac failure or ventricular arrhythmia or asymptomatic and be discovered incidentally by echocardiography. They regress spontaneously in the majority of cases as demonstrated in section 3 of the CD-ROM. They must be differentiated from hypertrophic cardiomyopathies and endocardial fibroelastosis. They are often multiple in tuberous sclerosis. When small, they can be difficult to recognize because of their intramural locations. On T1-weighted SE images rhabdomyomas may appear as medium or more often as high signal intensity masses not well demarcated from adjacent myocardium. The large tumors may occupy the entire cavity as in the case shown in Fig. 4.7. After gadolinium injection the rhabdomyomas show clear enhancement.

4.3 Primary Cardiac Tumors – Malignant Tumors

Primary malignant tumors of the heart are rare, comprising approximately one-third of all primary cardiac tumors. The most common primary cardiac malignancies are sarcomas, 33% being angiosarcomas, 20% rhabdomyosarcomas, 15% mesotheliomas, and about 10% being malignant fibrous histiocytomas [12,13].

4.3.1 Angiosarcoma

Angiosarcoma is the most commonly seen cardiac mass in men between 20 and 50 years of age, representing approximately 70% of the cardiac malignancies in this group. This tumor is more frequently located in the right atrium or the pericardium presenting symptoms related to inflow obstruction or pericardial constriction. This

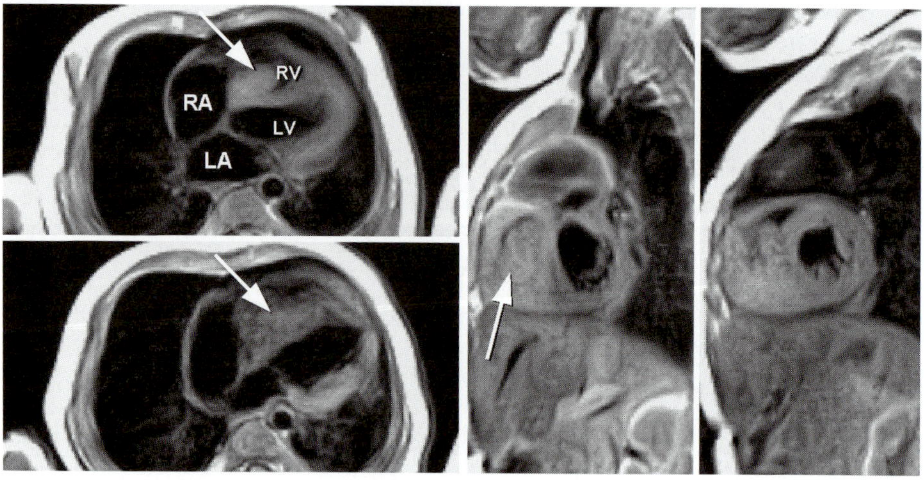

Fig. 4.7 Rhabdomyoma of the right ventricle.
Transverse T1w SE images show a huge right ventricular mass of medium signal intensity (arrow). The mass obstructs the entire right ventricular cavity.
RA = right atrium, LA = left atrium, LV = left ventricle.

tumor is highly malignant with dissemination of distant metastasis to the lungs, liver and lymph nodes [14,15].

Kaposi's sarcoma represents a subtype of angiosarcoma of the heart, which may occur as a primary cardiac neoplasm in patients with acquired immunodeficiency syndrome (AIDS).

4.3.2 Rhabdomyosarcoma and Fibrosarcoma

Primary sarcomas of the heart include rhabdomyosarcoma, fibrosarcoma and osteosarcoma. Rhabdomyosarcoma and osteosarcoma occur with equal incidence in the right and left sides of the heart, while osteosarcomas more commonly originate from the posterior wall of the left atrium. The shape and signal characteristics of these tumors on MR images can vary significantly [16].

4.3.3 Mesothelioma

Mesothelioma is a malignant tumor that originates from the pericardium and therefore the most common clinical presentation includes signs of pericardial constriction and right heart failure. Unlike pleural mesothelioma, a relationship to asbestos exposure has not been established. MR imaging is particularly useful for the evaluation of the extent and topology of the tumor as a well as the hemodynamic impact on the ventricular function [17].

4.3.4 Malignant Fibrous Histiocytoma

Malignant fibrous histiocytomas (MFH) consist of primitive mesenchymal and fibroblastic cells, and predominantly appear as a sessile tumor arising from the left atrium or the interatrial septum. About two-third of MFH are multiple and careful scrutiny of secondary lesions should always be undertaken. MR signal characteristics of MFH demonstrate intermediate T1 signal with slight heterogeneity and predominantly increased T2 signal [12, 18].

4.4 Secondary Cardiac Tumors

Secondary tumors of the heart are 20 to 40 times more frequent than primary tumors. The most common primary tumors are carcinomas of the lung (Fig. 4.**8**), breast, lymphoma, malignant melanoma, leukemia and extension of tumors of the upper abdomen such as carcinomas of the liver, of the kidneys and of the adrenals [10]. There are three modes of extension of the primary tumors to the heart: direct spread from lung and mediastinal tumors, venous invasion from tumors of the abdomen through the inferior vena cava and into the right atrium and by systemic metastasis to the pericardium, myocardium and cardiac cavities (Fig. 4.**9**). The diagnosis is easy when the primary tumor is discovered and extension demonstrated. The diagnosis can be more difficult when the secondary tumor is isolated [19]. In this case the goal

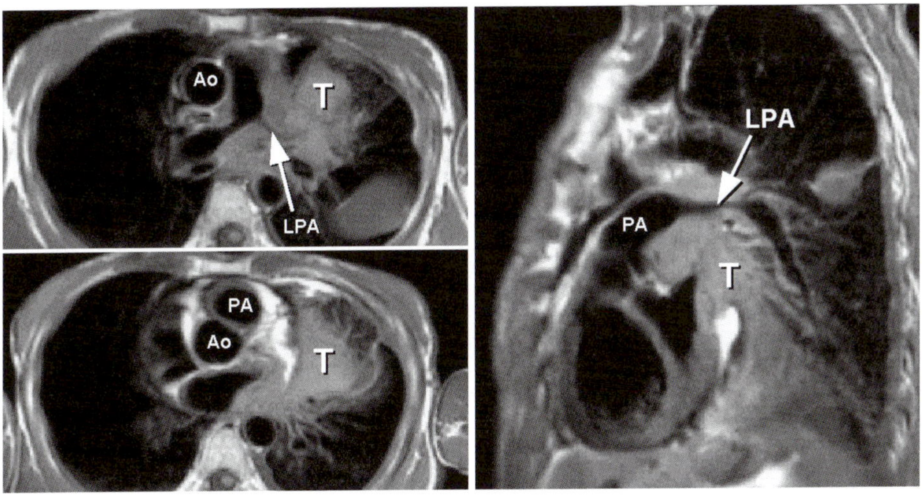

Fig. 4.**8** Bronchogenic carcinoma.
Transverse T1w SE images show an intermediate signal intensity mass (T) extending from the left hilum to the left atrium. After gadolinium injection there is massive enhancement of the mass (bottom left). Note severe compression and extension to both pulmonary arteries (arrow). Sagittal oblique T1w SE images confirmed the severe narrowing of the left pulmonary artery (LPA) and the extension of the intermediate signal intensity mass in the left atrium.

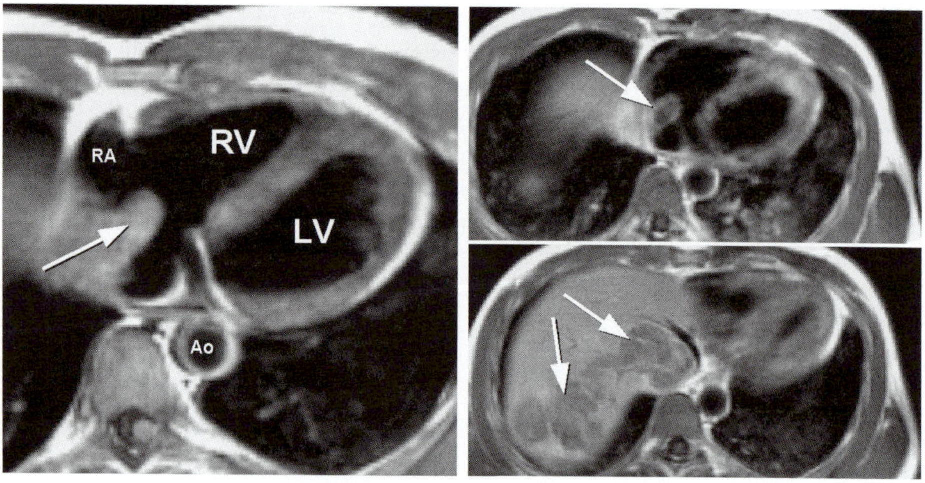

Fig. 4.**9** Atrial extension of hepatocarcinoma.
Transverse T1w SE images show an intermediate signal intensity mass (arrow) extending from the inferior vena cava to the right atrium.

Table 4.**1** MRI characteristics of common cardiac masses [modified from Bogaert J, et al. in: Magnetic Resonance of the heart and great vessels. Bogaert J, Duerinckx AJ, Rademakers FE (eds), Springer Verlag]

	intensity on T1 w SE	**intensity on cine GE**	**Gd Contrast Enhancement**
Benign cardiac tumors			
Myxoma	variable	low	yes
Lipoma & Lipomatus atrial septum	high	medium	no
Rhabdomyoma	medium	low	as myocardium
Fibroma	medium	low	variable
Hemangioma			
Malignant cardiac tumors			
Angiosarcoma	variable	low	yes
Rhabdomyosarcoma	medium	variable	yes
Lymphoma	medium	low	yes
Pericardial mesothelioma			
Non cardiac masses			
Thrombus	medium	low	no
Valvular vegetation	–	low	no
Hydatid cyst	low	high	no
Pleuropercardial cyst	low	high	no

is to differentiate tumor from thrombus, clot being the most frequent mass of the heart. This differentiation may be difficult using SE techniques. Thrombus may have variable signal intensity on SE images depending upon its age. Fresh thrombus may have medium-to-high signal intensity on T1-weighted images and bright signal on T2-weighted images. Chronic thrombus may have low signal intensity on both T1- and T2-weighted images. Tumors have usually medium signal intensity on T1-weighted images but may be variable as well. Most tumors have high signal intensity on T2-weighted images. Differentiation can be easier with cine-GE images where clots may have low signal intensity, but not always as demonstrated on Fig. 4.**11**, whereas tumors have medium signal intensity. The most reliable technique is the injection of gadolinium both in SE and cine-GE images. Tumor enhances with gadolinium whereas this enhancement is generally not seen in thrombus.

4.5 Non-Tumoral Cardiac Masses

4.5.1 Intracardiac Thrombi

The most common etiology for an intracardiac mass remains a thrombus. The first step in evaluation of an intracavitary mass is to differentiate true solid masses from slow blood flow artifacts [18]. This is particularly critical when both can coexist in the case of a large mass obstructing blood flow or in the case of infarction with decreased wall motion and adjacent slow flow and parietal thrombus [19]. There are several ways to differentiate a solid mass from slow flow:

1. Acquisition of phase-contrast images where the solid mass appears in gray as other adjacent structures whereas blood flow, even slow, appears in white or black depending on the flow direction.
2. Cine MRI sequences demonstrating high signal intensity of slow moving blood compared to medium or low intensity of solid masses (Fig. 4.**10**).

The next step is to differentiate tumor from thrombus. This differentiation may be difficult using SE techniques. Thrombus may have variable signal intensity on SE images depending upon its age. Fresh thrombus may have medium-to-high signal intensity on T1-weighted images and bright signal on T2-weighted images. Areas of bright and medium signal intensity can be associated in the mass. Chronic thrombus may have low signal intensity on both T1- and T2-weighted images. Cine gradient-echo (GE) images are more sensitive for the detection of intracardiac thrombi than SE images [20]. On GE images thrombi (except for hyperacute thrombi) show low contrast intensity compared to myocardium. Tumors, on the other hand, generally have increased signal intensity on GE images. Atrial myxoma is an exception, as this tumor typically appears as a low intensity structure on GE images. The most reliable technique for differentiating thrombi from tumors is the injection of gadolinium-DTPA both in SE and cine-GE images. Tumor enhances with gadolinium whereas this enhancement is generally not seen with thrombus (Fig. 4.**11**).

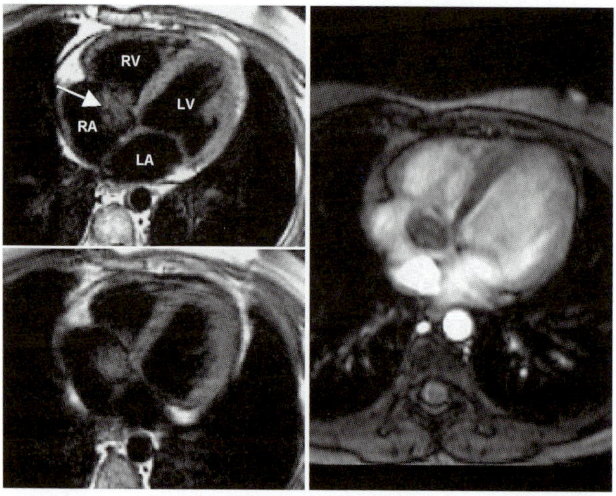

Fig. 4.**10** Thrombus in the right atrium.
Transverse T1w SE images (left) show an intermediate signal intensity mass extending from the extremity of the superior vena cava to the tricuspid valve (arrow). On cine gradient-echo image (right), the thrombus appears as a low signal intensity mass.
RA = right atrium, LA = left atrium, LV = left ventricle, RV = right ventricle.

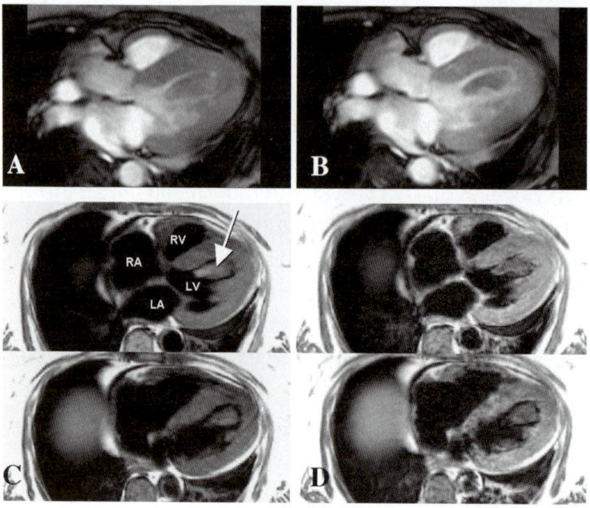

Fig. 4.**11** Thrombus in the left ventricle.
Cine gradient-echo (**A**) and T1w SE images (**C**) before and after (**B**, **D**) gadolinium injection show a symmetric hypertrophic cardiomyopathy and a mass (arrow) with a signal intensity higher than adjacent myocardium on SE images. After contrast injection a massive enhancement of the myocardium is demonstrated on both SE and GE images, whereas the mass remains with the same signal intensity.

4.5.2 Endocarditis and Valvular Vegetations

Bacterial endocarditis may be responsible for vegetation and destruction of a cardiac valve as well as abscess and pseudoaneurysms adjacent to the valve leaflets. MRI plays an important role in demonstrating and localizing the pseudoaneurysms complicating perivalvular abscesses particularly with the help of cine gradient-echo (GE) techniques which demonstrate flow in the pseudoaneurysm as well as associated turbulent flow due to valve stenosis or regurgitation [21]. On spin-echo (SE) images it can be difficult to see the cavity of the pseudoaneurysm because of slow flow and associated thrombus in the cavity. Vegetations are usually small and better detected by echocardiography. SE imaging is limited in depicting these small vegetations be-

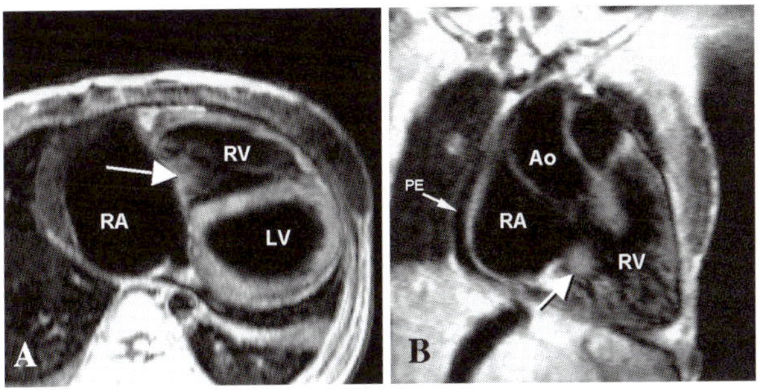

Fig. 4.12 Transverse and coronal T1w SE images show severe enlargement of right cavities, pericardial effusion (PE) and an intermediate signal intensity mass (arrow) at the level of the tricuspid valve.
RA = right atrium, RV = right ventricle, LV = left ventricle, Ao =aorta.

cause it can be difficult to differentiate them from flow artifacts. Associated calcifications may also appear as a signal loss. On the other hand, cine GE techniques can detect small vegetations which appear as low or intermediate signal intensity in bright flowing blood. Huge vegetations as in the case shown in Fig. 4.12, may be detected on SE images as well as on cine images. Because of the composition of the vegetation with fibrosis and organized fibrinopurulent tissue it is usually impossible to differentiate it from a thrombus. Furthermore, its signal usually does not increase after gadolinium injection. Cine images are particularly useful in the assessment of associated valve dysfunctions. For example, cine MRI was the only method demonstrating a flow void due to the rupture of the sinus of Valsalva in the right ventricle (see CD ROM for dynamic cine images of that case).

4.5.3 Hydatid Cysts

Hydatid cyst is a parasitic disease due to development of the larva of the tapeworm *Echinococcus granulosus*. The liver is the organ the most frequently involved. Cardiac infestation is rare and the most frequent site of development is the left ventricular wall via the left coronary artery. Severe arrhythmia is one mode of clinical presentation. Sudden death may occur due to rupture into the pericardium and tamponade. CT scan is superior to MRI in demonstrating calcifications in the cyst. On MR images they appear as low signal intensity foci within the mass [22]. On T1-weighted images hydatid cyst appears as medium to high signal intensity mass depending upon its content. It can be homogeneous and surrounded by a low signal intensity rim or heterogeneous with the presence of partitions due to several cysts and daughter cysts. On T2-weighted images high signal intensity is typical of fluid collection. After gadolinium injection there is usually no enhancement (Fig. 4.13).

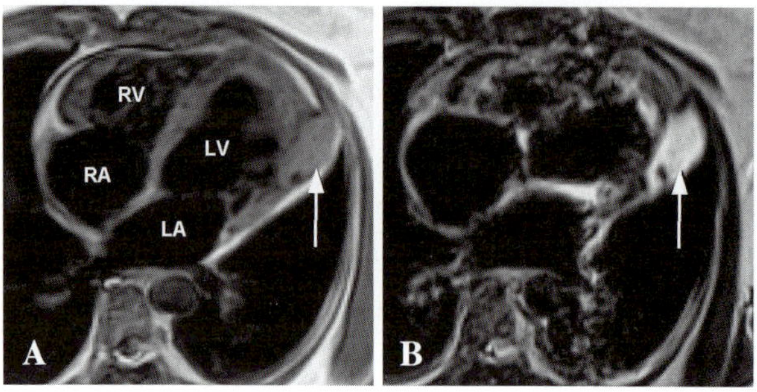

Fig. 4.**13** Hydatic cyst. Transverse T1w SE image after gadolinium injection (**A**). There is no enhancement of the mass (arrow). T2w SE image (**B**) shows high signal intensity of the mass demonstrating its liquid content. Calcifications within the cyst appear as low signal intensity.

4.6 References

1. Martin DR, Merchant N, MacDonald C. MR imaging of cardiac masses: A review of current applications and approach. Applied Radiology 2000; 5: 10–20.
2. Bogaert J. Cardiac Masses. In: Magnetic Resonance of the Heart and Great Vessels. Bogaert J, Duerinckx AJ, Rademakers FE (eds), Springer Verlag, Heidelberg, 1999.
3. Araoz P, Mulvagh S, Tazelaar H., Julsrud P, Breen J. CT and MR imaging of benign primary cardiac neoplasms with echocardiographic correlation. RadioGraphics 2000; 20: 1303–1319.
4. Matsuoka H, Hamada M, Honda T, et al. Morphologic and histologic characterization of cardiac myxomas by magnetic resonance imaging. Angiology 1996; 47: 693–698.
5. de Roos A, Weijers E, van Duinen S, Van der Wall EE. Calcified right atrial myxoma demonstrated by magnetic resonance imaging. 1989; Chest 95: 478–479.
6. Watanabe M, Takazawa K, Wada A, et al. Cardiac myxoma with gamna-Gandy bodies: case report with MR imaging. J Thorac Imaging 1994; 9: 185–187.
7. Obeid AI, Marvasti M, Parker F, Rosenberg J. Comparison of transthoracic and transesophageal echocardiography in diagnosis of left atrial myxoma. Am J Cardiol 1989; 63: 1006–1008.
8. Hananouchi GI, Goff WB. Cardiac lipoma. Six-year follow-up with MRI characteristics, and a review of the literature. Magn Reson Imaging 1990; 8: 825–828.
9. Kozelj M, Angelski A, Pavcnik D. Lipomatous hypertrophy of the interatrial septum: Diagnosis by echocardiography and magnetic resonance imaging, A case report. Angiology 1995; 46: 863–866.
10. Lund JT, Ehman AL, Julsrud PA, et al. Cardiac masses: Assessment by MR imaging. AJR Am J Roentgenol 1989; 152: 469–473.
11. Beghetti M, Gow AM, Haney I, et al. Pediatric primary benign cardiac tumors: A 15-year review. Am Heart J 1997; 134:1107–1114.
12. Kim EE, Wallace S, Abello A, et al. Malignant cardiac fibrous histiocytomas and angiosarcomas: MR features. J Comput Assist Tomogr 1989; 13: 627–632.
13. Siripornpitak S, Higgins CB. MRI of primary malignant cardiovascular tumors. J Comput Assist Tomogr 1997; 21: 462–466.

14. Aaaf HN, Aaaf JH. Sarcomas related to the heart and vasculature. Semin Surg Oncol 1994; 10: 374–382.
15. Naka N, Ohsawa M, Tomita Y, Kanno H, Uchida A, Aozasa K. Angiosarcoma in Japan. Cancer 1995; 75: 989–996.
16. Szucs RA, Rehr RB, Yanovich S, Tatum IL. Magnetic resonance imaging of cardiac rhabdomyosarcoma. Quantifying the response to chemotherapy. Cancer 1991; 67: 2066–2070.
17. Kaminaga T, Yamada N, Imakita S, Takamiya M, Nishimura T. Magnetic resonance imaging of pericardial malignant mesothelioma. Magn Reson Imaging 1993; 11: 1057–1061.
18. Catton C, Shulman H, Austhoven J, Wilk A. Gated magnetic resonance imaging of metastatic intracardiac malignant fibrous histiocytoma. Can Assoc Radiol J 1990; 41; 96–97.
19. Geibel A, Kasper W, Keck A, et al. Diagnosis, localization and evaluation of malignancy of heart and mediastinal tumors by conventional and transesophageal echocardiography. Acta Cardiol 1996; 51: 395–408.
20. Semelka AC, Shoenut JP, Wilson ME, et al. Cardiac masses: Signal intensity features on spin-echo, gradient-echo, gadolinium-enhanced spin-echo, and TurboFLASH images. J Magn Reson Imaging 1992; 2: 415–420.
21. Gomes AS, Lois JF, Child JS, et al. Cardiac tumors and thrombus: Evaluation with MR imaging. AJR Am J Roentgenol 1987; 149: 895–899.
22. Jungehulsing M, Sechtem U, Theissen P, Hilger HH, Schicha H. Left ventricular thrombi: evaluation with spin-echo and gradient-echo MR imaging. Radiology 1992; 182: 225–229.
23. Caduff JH, Hernandez RI, Ludomirsky A. MR visualization of aortic valve vegetations. Comput Assist Tomogr 1996; 20: 613–615.
24. Murayama S, Murakami J, Watanabe H, et al. Signal intensity characteristics of mediastinal cystic masses on T1-weighted MRI. J Comput Assist Tomogr 1995; 19: 188–191.

5 Valvular Heart Disease

Color Doppler echocardiography has significantly modified the strategy for the evaluation of valvular heart disease [1–4]. It often provides the complete information required for planning surgery. Furthermore, anatomic information with regard to leaflet number, valvular thickness and the presence of vegetations in endocarditis remain best provided by echocardiography. Invasive techniques such as cardiac catheterization are usually limited to the preoperative evaluation of the coronary arteries, as well as for quantitative measurements of cardiac hemodynamics or when there are discrepancies between clinical findings and echocardiographic data [5]. Recent reports and studies have demonstrated that MR imaging can be envisioned as an attractive alternative or a technique complementary to echocardiography [6–9]. This non-invasive technique provides three-dimensional, anatomic and functional data as well as potentially more accurate and more reproducible measurements of ventricular function than echocardiography [10]. The velocity-encoded MR (VEC-MR) imaging technique allows accurate estimation of velocity profiles across a valve or any vascular structure, thus providing sometimes more precise quantitative results than Doppler echocardiography [11,12]. Furthermore, MR imaging does not encounter the same limitations and problems of acoustic penetration for accessing different portions of the heart and, therefore, may provide a better visualization of morphology and flow velocity throughout the cardiovascular structures.

This chapter reviews existing MR imaging techniques used to evaluate valvular heart disease and discusses the advantages and limitations of these techniques for providing clinically useful information in cardiac valvular disease. For a detailed description of the different imaging techniques, see the first chapter of this book and for examples of dynamic images of selected valvular heart diseases cases, see the fourth section in the companion CD-ROM.

5.1 Imaging Techniques

The different imaging techniques used for the evaluation of valvular heart diseases comprise: spin-echo and/or fast spin-echo, cine gradient-echo and other fast cine imaging techniques and flow-sensitive imaging techniques.

5.1.1 Spin-Echo and Fast Spin-Echo Techniques

Spin-echo images may in some cases allow partial visualization of some valve anomalies such as thickening of the leaflets or bicuspid valve. However, this technique is particularly suitable to demonstrate the morphological changes in cardiac anatomy that are consequences of valvular disease such as enlargement or hypertrophy of cardiac chambers or distortions of aortic and pulmonary vessels.

5.1.2 Cine MR Imaging

The dynamic "cine-MR" imaging techniques are commonly used to acquire multi-frame sequences of a typical average cardiac cycle. Commonly, a minimum of 16 frames is necessary to adequately evaluate motion and function occurring in the complete cardiac cycle. The distribution of frames along the cardiac cycle must be set to allow full coverage of the R-R interval with the last frame of the series being as close as possible to the next R. The cine imaging sequences are particularly suitable for evaluating cardiac function and for identifying abnormal flow patterns encountered in valve disease.

For evaluation of cardiac function, the images are acquired in standardized planes referred to as horizontal long axis, vertical long axis and short axis. These standard planes, previously described in Chapter 1 [13], are positioned parallel to the long axis of the heart for the two first ones and perpendicular to the long axis for the short axis one.

On standard cine image sequences, blood has bright signal intensity and abnormal flow patterns encountered in valvular disease cause dephasing of the spins within a voxel and result in a signal loss (flow void). This signal void, present either in stenosis or regurgitation, is caused by high velocity flow and turbulence [14]. In gradient-echo (GE) cine imaging techniques it has been demonstrated previously that this flow void is dependent upon technical factors: the display parameters (window width and window level), the flip angle and particularly the echo time [15]. With a long echo time the signal void is well demonstrated whereas with short TE it tends to disappear (see Chapter 1). This dependency must be taken into account when evaluating flow anomalies in valve diseases.

One way to decrease acquisition time considerably with cine-GE technique is to use segmentation of the k space. This technique allows the reduction of the imaging time by a factor of 2 or 3 depending on the heart rate while keeping an adequate spatial resolution.

Fast GRE pulse sequences with a typical TR value of 4 to 8 milliseconds and TE equal to 2 to 4 milliseconds have recently been used, allowing cine-images to be acquired within a single breath-hold, thus eliminating respiratory artifacts. These sequences are less suitable to evaluate flow anomalies encountered in valvular heart disease because of the short TE employed but are ideal to evaluate cardiac wall motion abnormalities, as well as for calculation of ventricular volumes, ejection fraction and cardiac mass [16].

5.1.3 Flow-Sensitive Imaging Techniques

Currently, the most popular flow-sensitive cine-MR technique used is the phase change technique based on the principle that the phase of flowing spins relative to stationary spins along a magnetic gradient changes in direct proportion to the velocity of flow. This technique, referred to as phase contrast, phase shift MR imaging or velocity-encoded cine MR imaging (VEC-MRI) allows quantification of blood velocity profiles at different points during the cardiac cycle [11,17,18]. Images can be reconstructed in magnitude, providing anatomic information and in phase, providing flow velocity information. The phase shift, proportional to the velocity, is displayed as variations in pixel intensity on the phase map image. Stationary tissue appears in gray whereas flow in the positive or negative direction along the flow-encoding axis will appear as bright or dark pixels, respectively. Thus, one can differentiate antegrade from retrograde flow [19]. Velocity can be encoded either on planes perpendicular to the direction of flow by using slice-selective direction (through-plane velocity measurement) or parallel to the direction of flow by using phased-encoded or frequency-encoded directions (in-plane velocity measurement) or more recently in three dimensions. However, VEC-MRI has potential sources of error and limitations [20] as already described in Chapter 1.

VEC-MRI can be used to calculate absolute velocity at each point in the cardiac cycle at given locations in the plane of data acquisition. The velocity can be measured for each pixel or within a region of interest (ROI) encircling the entire or parts of the vessel cross-sectional area or across a valve annulus. Based on the measurement of the cross-sectional area on the magnitude image, the product of area and spatial mean velocity (average value for all pixels in the cross-sectional area on the phase image) yields instantaneous flow volume for a specific time frame in the cardiac cycle. Integration of all instantaneous flow volumes throughout the cardiac cycle gives the volume flow per heartbeat. This technique has been evaluated in vitro as well as in vivo by several authors to yield accurate measurements of aortic and pulmonary artery flow, representing the stroke volumes of the left ventricle and the right ventricle, respectively [21,22]. These measurements are applied to the evaluation and quantitative assessment of regurgitant as well as stenotic valvular lesions.

5.2 Quantitative Analysis Techniques

5.2.1 Detection and Quantification of a Valvular Regurgitation

There are three methods to evaluate the severity of valvular regurgitation:

1. Measurement of the area of signal void.
2. Regurgitant fraction calculated with ventricular volumetric measurements.
3. Quantification of the regurgitant blood flow by velocity-encoded cine MR (VEC-MR).

5.2.1.1 Measurement of the Area of Signal Void

Cine gradient-echo (GE) images can be used for evaluation of the severity of valvular regurgitation based on the area or the volume of the signal void encountered in an insufficient valve. Mitral regurgitation is identified as a signal loss coming from the insufficient mitral valve into the left atrium during ventricular systole whereas aortic regurgitation is identified as a signal loss extending from the incompetent aortic valve into the left ventricle during ventricular diastole [23].

The regurgitant jets are three-dimensional structures and these abnormal jets are different from one patient to another, depending upon the type of valvular alteration. Thus, the imaging plane may influence the apparent size of the signal loss and more than one plane is recommended to evaluate its size [14]. Based on the same qualitative gradings used for Doppler echocardiography, cine-GE imaging allows objective assessment of the severity of a valvular regurgitation by several measurements [24,25].

1. Area or volume of the signal void in the receiving cavity.
2. Maximum length of the signal void in the receiving cavity.
3. Ratio of the area of signal void to the area of the chamber receiving the regurgitant jet.

However, it has been demonstrated that the measurements of dimensions of the signal void with cine-GE technique are only semiquantitative indices of the severity of regurgitation [7,24,25].

Among the different frames acquired during a R-R interval, the image on which the signal loss shows the largest size is used for the measurement (Fig. 5.1). The signal loss is usually outlined manually and can be significantly different depending on the

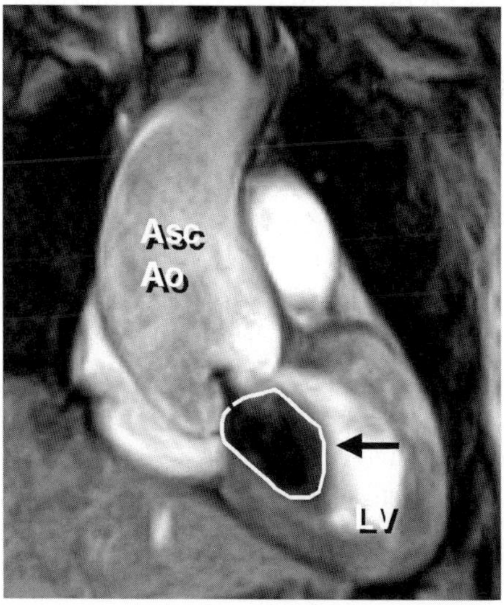

Fig. 5.1 Example of the measurement of the area of signal void (arrow) on cine-GE images in aortic regurgitation (coronal view) allowing assessment of the severity of the valvular regurgitation. The frame on which the signal loss shows the largest size is used for this measurement. After appropriate adjustment of the image display settings (window level and window size), manual tracing of the edges of the area of signal void is performed. The resulting outlines of the area of signal void and the chosen image settings remain subjective and can vary between observers.
Asc Ao = ascending aorta, LV = left ventricle.

image display settings (window level and width). The resulting outlines of the signal void are subjective and can therefore vary significantly between observers. Thus, this method has limitations due to technical factors, as mentioned above, particularly the echo time and the display parameters and due to physiopathologic factors (changes in volume and pressure of the receiving cavity can result in significant alterations in the distribution of the regurgitant jet) [15]. Furthermore, the regurgitant jets are 3D structures that change shape and direction throughout the cardiac cycle.

5.2.1.2 Regurgitant Fraction Calculated with Ventricular Volumetric Measurements

Ventricular volumes can be estimated from cine-GE images either on horizontal long axis (4 chamber view), vertical long axis (2 chamber view) and/or several short axis views of the ventricles. Depending upon the acquisition planes available, one can apply different formulas validated in echocardiography by measuring area (A) and length (L) of the cavities. The most practical approach for measuring volumes is to use the simplified Simpson formula by using 2 short axis planes and the 4 chamber view where the area of the ventricles is measured on the short axis views and the length of the cavity is measured on the 4 chamber view (Figs 5.**2** and 5.**3**) [13]. The formula can be expressed as:

$$V = \frac{L}{2}(A_{MV} + \frac{2}{3}A_{PM}),$$

where L is the length of the ventricle, A_{MV} represents the area of the ventricle on the slice obtained just below the mitral valve, and A_{PM} the area of the ventricle on the slice obtained at the level of the papillary muscles. In normal hearts the right ventricular stroke volume (RV Str V) and left ventricular stroke volume (LV Str V) are equal. The ventricular stroke volume is the difference between the end-diastolic volume (usually calculated on the first image after the R wave) and the end-systolic volume (calculated on the image with the smallest ventricular area). The difference in stroke volume between a regurgitant ventricle (LV in mitral and aortic regurgitation) and a normal ventricle (right ventricle) is the regurgitant volume (RegV). The regurgitant fraction (RF) can be calculated as the RegV divided by the Str V of the regurgitant ventricle. RF has been used to evaluate the severity of regurgitation: mild: RF = 15–20%, moderate: RF = 20–40%, severe: RF > 40% [26]. One limitation of this method is that the formulas used for the measurement of the ventricular volumes apply well for the left ventricle which has an elliptic shape but less well for the right ventricle. Another limitation is that it cannot be applied in cases of multivalvular disease. If there is coexistence of mitral and aortic regurgitations, the total volume of regurgitation will be calculated and if regurgitation exists on both sides of the heart (mitral and tricuspid regurgitations) the calculation will be meaningless.

Another way to calculate stroke volumes of the right and left ventricles is to use VEC-MR by measuring flow in the ascending aorta and pulmonary artery on a plane perpendicular to the vessel [22]. Flow is the product of the mean velocity in the vessel

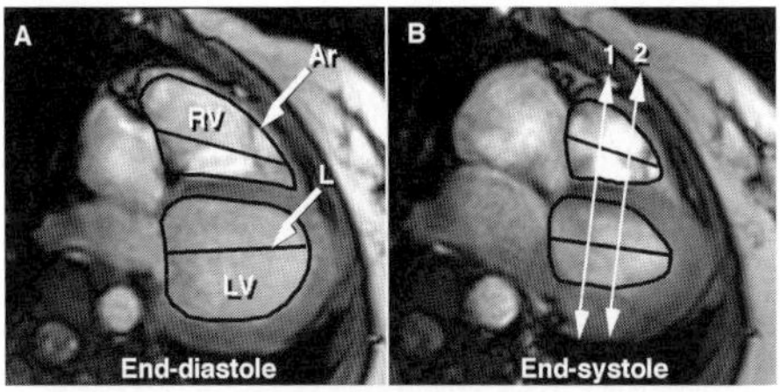

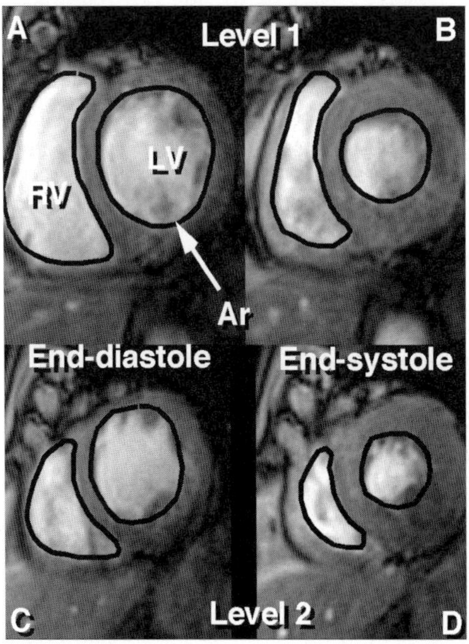

Figs. 5.**2** and 5.**3** Regurgitant fraction calculated with ventricular volumetric measurements on cine-GE images.
Ventricular volumes can be calculated either on long axis images (four chamber view) (Fig. 5.**2**) or short axis images of the ventricles (Fig. 5.**3**). Depending upon the acquisition planes available, one can apply different formulas by measuring area (Ar) and length (L) of the cavities (see text). On Fig. 5.**2B**, the planes are positioned perpendicular to the long axis of the ventricles to perform short axis levels 1 and 2 (double arrows 1 and 2). End-diastolic volumes are calculated on the first image after the R wave whereas end-systolic volumes are calculated on the image with the smallest ventricular area. The stroke volume is the difference between the end-diastolic volume and the end-systolic volume. The difference in stroke volume between the regurgitant ventricle (left ventricle in mitral and aortic regurgitation) and the normal ventricle (right ventricle) is the regurgitant volume. Regurgitant fraction is the regurgitant volume divided by the stroke volume of the regurgitant ventricle.
RV = right ventricle, LV= left ventricle.

and the area of the vessel on each time frame during the cardiac cycle. Integration of the flow for all images during systole provides a measurement of the systolic flow. Thus, stroke volumes of the left ventricle and the right ventricle can be calculated respectively.

5.2.1.3 Quantification of the Regurgitant Blood Flow by Velocity-Encoded Cine MR (VEC-MR)

VEC-MR allows quantification of blood velocity profiles by generating a flow velocity map where moving blood appears in black or white, depending upon the direction of flow (antegrade or retrograde) whereas stationary tissue appears in gray (Fig. 5.**4**) [27,28]. Consequently, retrograde flow can be identified and quantified.

The cardiac cycle is usually segmented into 16 frames equally spaced. For each frame, the cross-sectional area (A) is measured from a region of interest (ROI) manually positioned around the vascular structure of interest (aorta, pulmonary artery,

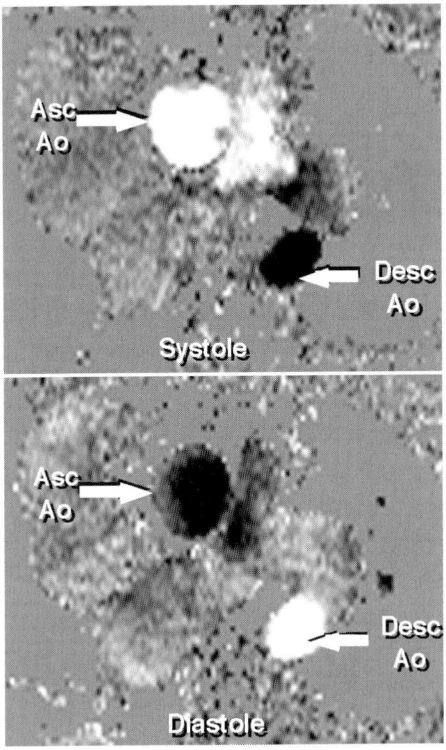

Fig. 5.**4** Transverse oblique VEC-MR phase images perpendicular to blood flow direction in the ascending aorta (Asc Ao) at the level of the right pulmonary artery in systole (top) and in diastole (bottom; seventh image of the sixteen frames performed) in a case of aortic regurgitation. Bright signal in the Asc Ao during systole indicates antegrade flow (arrow) whereas dark signal in the Asc Ao during diastole indicates retrograde flow (arrow). Opposite signals are seen in the descending aorta (Desc Ao). Stationary tissue appears in gray. The vessel must be outlined on magnitude images and then transferred on these phase images because the edges of the vessel appear in gray as surrounding stationary tissue at end-diastole. The region of interest (ROI) traced on the magnitude image is transferred on the corresponding phase image for each frame, allowing through-plane measurement of the average velocity (AvV). The product of the area measured on the magnitude image and AvV in the ROI gives the instantaneous flow at each time frame. Integration of flow values for each frame estimates blood flow volumes per heartbeat.

mitral and tricuspid annulus) on the magnitude images. Then, this ROI is transferred from the magnitude image to the corresponding phase image for each frame, thus allowing measurement of the average velocity (AvV). The product of A and AvV in the ROI gives the instantaneous flow at each time frame. Integration of flow values for each frame estimates blood flow volumes. Because the area of the vessel is a squared value and because this area changes during the cardiac cycle, a precise measurement of the cross-sectional area must be obtained on the magnitude image at each time frame of the cardiac cycle before transferring the ROI onto the corresponding phase image. The technique allows one to distinguish between antegrade and retrograde flow so that flow below zero line corresponding to retrograde flow can be calculated by measuring the area bounded by the curve under the baseline which represents the regurgitant volume (Fig. 5.**5**). Measurements must not be performed at the site of the incompetent valve because of the presence of artifacts, eddy currents and complex motion of the valve through the imaging plane but proximal or distal to the valve annulus (aorta at the level of right pulmonary artery for aortic regurgitation).

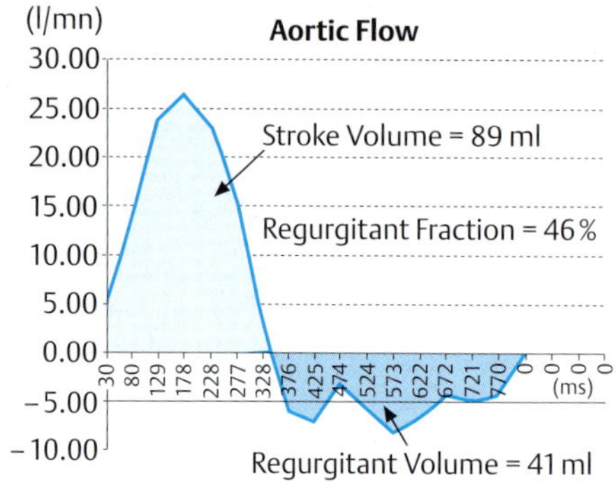

Fig. 5.**5** Flow volume curve versus time in the ascending aorta of a patient with aortic regurgitation. The area (light blue) under the initial positive part of the curve in systole represents the stroke volume. The latter part of the curve below the baseline (dark blue) represents the retrograde flow in diastole. Regurgitant volume is calculated as the area bounded by the curve under the baseline during diastole. The regurgitant fraction, which is defined as regurgitant volume divided by the stroke volume, has been calculated to 46% that indicates a severe aortic regurgitation.

5.2.2 Detection and Quantification of a Valvular Stenosis

There are two methods to evaluate the severity of valvular stenosis:

1. Evaluation of the flow jet and associated findings and direct measurement of the valve area.
2. Quantification of transvalvular pressure gradient and valve area by velocity-encoded cine MR (VEC-MR).

5.2.2.1 Evaluation of the Flow Jet and Associated Findings

Cine-GE images can be used for grading the severity of valvular stenosis based on the size and extent of the abnormal flow jet [29] (signal void caused by high-velocity flow and turbulence) and associated findings (valve leaflet thickening, reduced valve motion, chamber enlargement and/or wall thickening) encountered in a stenotic valve.

Mitral stenosis is identified as a signal loss coming from the mitral valve into the left ventricle during ventricular diastole whereas aortic stenosis is identified as a signal loss extending from the aortic valve into the ascending aorta during ventricular systole (Fig. 5.**6**).

The abnormal motion of the stenotic valve can be evaluated on a plane parallel to the annulus, particularly on short TE images such as the magnitude images obtained with VEC-MR technique. The valve area can also often be measured directly on these magnitude images of the VEC-MR sequence because on these short TE sequences the flow void caused by the stenosis is not detected (Fig. 5.**7**). This measurement was shown to correlate well with Doppler echocardiography and catheterization [30].

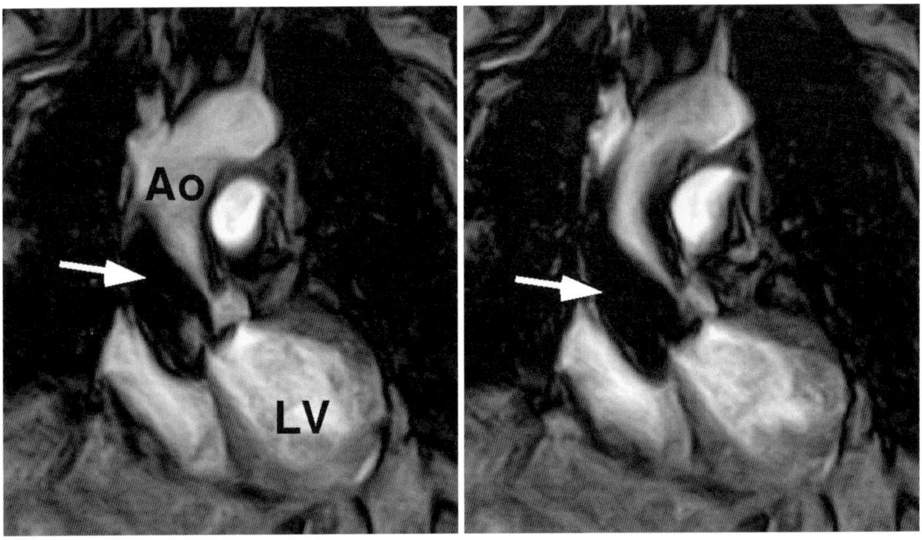

Fig. 5.6 Coronal cine-GE images at the early systole (left) and at midsystole (right) of a patient with tight valvular aortic stenosis. The area and the extent of the signal loss (arrow) due to acceleration and turbulent flow give a qualitative evaluation of the degree of the stenosis.
Ao = aorta, LV = left ventricle.

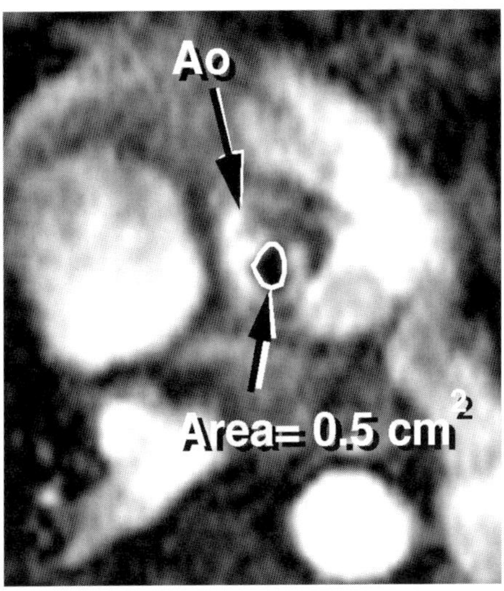

Fig. 5.7 Transverse axial cine-GE image (magnitude image of the VEC-MR sequence) parallel to the aortic annulus (Ao) allows the direct measurement of the valve area. The use of short TE sequence as in the magnitude image of the VEC-MR sequence decreases the appearance of the flow void and allows evaluation of the abnormal motion of the stenotic valve as well as calculation of the valve area, in this case 0.5 cm^2.

5.2.2.2 Quantification of Transvalvular Pressure Gradient and Valve Area by Velocity-Encoded Cine MR (VEC-MR)

VEC-MR allows quantification of stenotic valves by measuring directly the increase of flow velocity in the jet of blood passing though the stenosis [12]. The measurement of the peak velocity or maximum velocity (V_{max}) within the stenotic jet can be obtained either on planes perpendicular to the direction of flow (through-plane velocity measurement) or parallel to the direction of flow (in-plane velocity measurement) (Figs. 5.**8** and 5.**9**). In-plane imaging usually provides sufficient pixels for analysis of velocity because the entire abnormal jet is displayed. But in case of very tight stenosis, where the jet is narrowed, in-plane measurement may be less reliable because of partial volume averaging and motion of the jet out of the imaging plane. Conversely, with through-plane imaging, only a slice of the jet is displayed and, depending upon the position of this slice within the jet, one can miss the true maximum velocity if the plane is too far from the valve orifice and it can lead to misregistration of flow due to signal loss resulting from turbulence and eddy currents if the plane is too close to the valve. Thus, it is preferable to measure data in both in- and through-planes [20]. The technical considerations are less demanding for the measurement of velocities less than 4 m/sec but for velocities up to 6 m/sec the use of short TE sequence (TE = 3–4 ms) is mandatory to improve the reliability and accuracy of the measurements [31]. The pressure gradient (ΔP) across the stenotic valve can be derived using the modified Bernoulli equation:

$$\Delta P = 4 \cdot (V_{max})^2$$

where ΔP is the pressure drop across the stenosis and V_{max} the peak velocity in m/sec measured in the stenotic jet.

The valve area (A Ao) can be calculated as well by using the continuity equation:

$$A\ Ao = A\ OT \times VOT/V\ Ao$$

where A OT is the outflow tract area, V OT is the maximum velocity in the outflow tract and V Ao is the maximum velocity measured within the stenotic jet [32]. It will be performed on planes parallel to the direction of flow (long axis in a stenotic aortic valve) (Fig. 5.**8**).

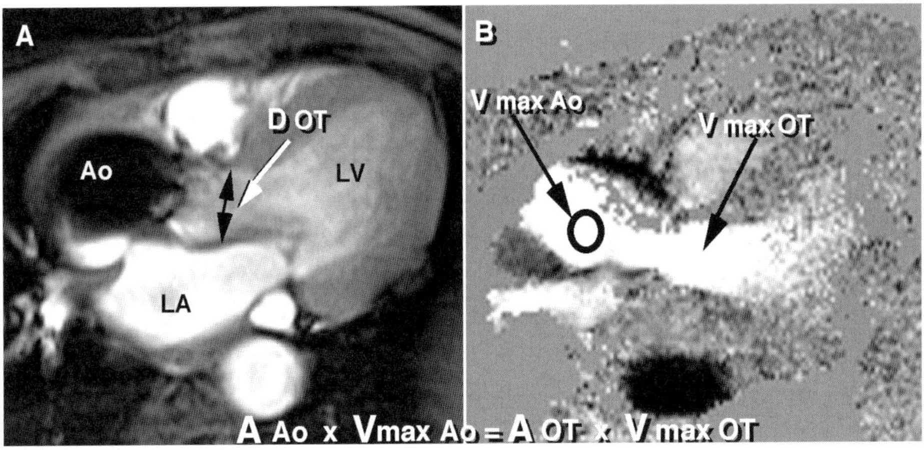

Fig. 5.**8** Long axis cine-GE image (**A**) and corresponding phase VEC-MR image (**B**) of a patient with severe aortic stenosis. The flow void corresponding to the stenotic jet in the ascending aorta (Ao) is well demonstrated on the cine-GE image. The calculation of the peak velocity (V_{max} Ao) can be performed by placing a ROI on a plane parallel to the direction of flow (in-plane velocity measurement) with velocity encoded left-to-right. In this plane, the calculation of the valve area can be performed as well by using the continuity equation.

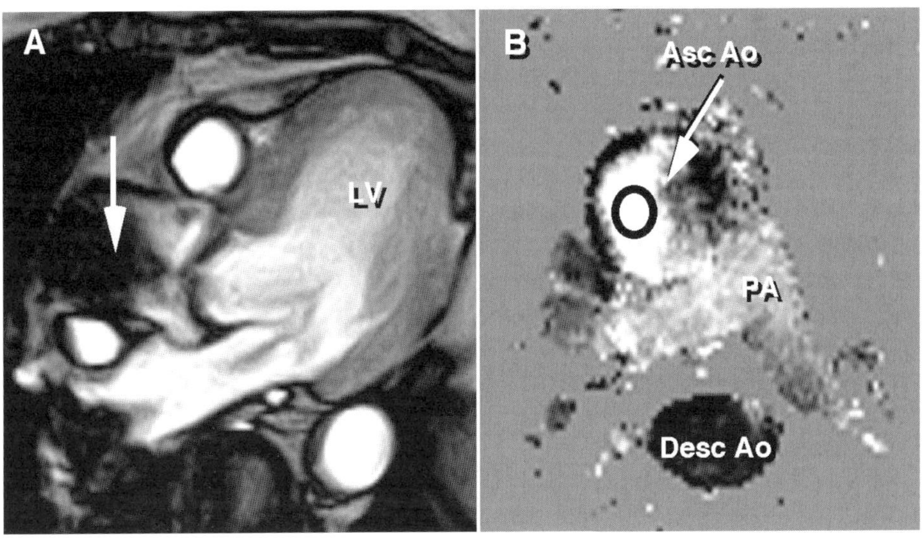

Fig. 5.**9** Long axis cine-GE image (**A**) and phase VEC-MR image (**B**) perpendicular to the direction of flow (through-plane velocity measurement) of a patient with aortic stenosis. The flow void corresponding to the stenotic jet in the ascending aorta (Ao) is well demonstrated on the cine-GE image (arrow). The calculation of the peak velocity (V_{max} Ao) can also be performed by placing a ROI within the stenotic jet in the ascending aorta (Asc Ao).
LV = left ventricle, PA = pulmonary artery.

5.3 Clinical Applications

5.3.1 Aortic Stenosis

Aortic stenosis is defined as a condition in which opening of the aortic valve in systole is restricted. It can be due to a variety of disorders that affect the cusps and/or annulus. In infants, children and young adults the major causes of aortic stenosis are congenital malformation of the cusps (bicuspid aortic valve) or annulus and rheumatic disease. Over 60 years of age the major causes are calcification of a bicuspid aortic valve and degeneration of valve cusps or annulus.

Spin-echo images can demonstrate thickening and bulging of the cusps, dilatation of ascending aorta (due to jet lesion) usually situated on the right border of the ascending aorta and left ventricular hypertrophy. In severe long-standing disease the left ventricle may enlarge. Cine-GE images can be used for evaluation of the severity of valvular stenosis based on the size and extent of the abnormal flow jet in the aorta (Fig. 5.**6**) and associated findings (valve leaflets thickening and bulging, reduced valve motion, chamber enlargement and/or wall thickening of the left ventricle) encountered in stenotic aortic valve. The optimal planes for identifying the signal void corresponding to the abnormal flow jet are the coronal plane centered on the left ventricular outflow tract and the long axis of the left ventricle (Figs. 5.**6**, 5.**8**, and 5.**9**).

The best method for evaluating aortic stenosis is through the calculation of the maximum velocity (V_{max}) within the stenotic jet. These measurements must be carried out both on planes perpendicular (Fig. 5.**8**) and parallel to the direction of flow (Fig. 5.**9**) as described previously [20]. Either a large ROI encompassing the entire jet or small ROI's at different locations within the jet, are positioned to measure the maximum velocity in the jet during peak systole. When the stenosis is tight, very high velocity jets are encountered and aortic annulus tends to be more horizontal. As in Doppler echocardiography, the pressure gradient across the stenotic valve can be calculated using the modified Bernoulli equation [32].

The valve area (A Ao) can be calculated as well by using the continuity equation described previously. Measurements of pressure gradient and valve area with VEC-MR technique corresponded well with data obtained from cardiac catheterization and Doppler echocardiography. But VEC-MRI has some advantages over Doppler echocardiography, particularly when the acoustic window is limited and in cases of complex flow patterns that are better demonstrated by MRI which displays the entire abnormal flow jet [32].

5.3.2 Aortic Regurgitation

Aortic regurgitation can be due to aortic cusp abnormalities, lesions of the annulus and dilatation of the aortic root. The most frequent causes are rheumatic disease, aortoannular ectasia, endocarditis or aortic root dilatation due to hypertension. Acute

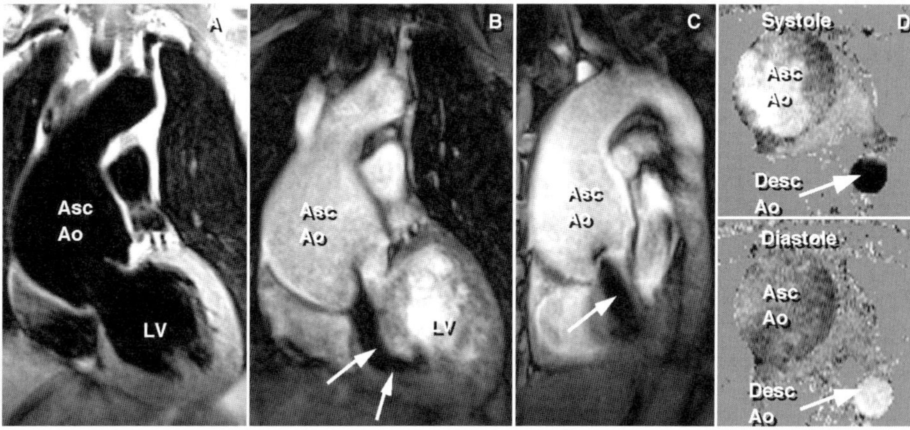

Fig. 5.**10** Coronal spin-echo image (**A**), coronal (**B**) and oblique sagittal (**C**) cine-GE images and transverse phase VEC-MR images (**D**) at the level of the ascending aorta (Asc Ao) in systole (top) and diastole (bottom) of a patient with severe aortic regurgitation. A large and long signal void is clearly visible on cine-GE images, extending from the incompetent aortic valve into the left ventricle (LV) in diastole (arrows) on both planes. Note the uniform massive dilatation of the aortic annulus and proximal ascending aorta (Ao) compatible with aortoannular ectasia. VEC-MR images permitted the calculation of a regurgitant fraction equal to 65%.

aortic regurgitation can be due to endocarditis, trauma or aortic dissection. The major hemodynamic consequence of aortic regurgitation is an increase of end-diastolic volume of the left ventricle. The need for surgery is determined by the severity of symptoms but more precise measurements of the degree of regurgitation and ventricular function are important as well. Doppler echocardiography and cardiac scintigraphy are usually used to assess left ventricular function as well as the degree of regurgitation non-invasively. However, color Doppler flow mapping evaluation is semiquantitative (measurement of jet length and width) and may be affected by several technical limitations. In cardiac scintigraphy, the degree of regurgitation is assessed by the difference between right and left ventricular stroke volumes. However, accuracy of stroke volume determination may be affected by superimposition of cardiac chambers and this method is only valid in isolated valvular regurgitation. Cardiac catheterization and angiography remain the gold standards in the assessment of the severity of aortic regurgitation and is still needed for evaluation of coronary arteries at present time. However, it is invasive, grading of regurgitation remains imprecise and underestimation of the degree of regurgitation may occur in severe regurgitation. Therefore, there is a need for a non-invasive method capable of direct measurement of regurgitant volume as well as ventricular function and MRI can play this role [32].

The etiology of aortic regurgitation can be assessed as for the case illustrated in Fig. 5.**10** where there is uniform dilatation of the aortic annulus and proximal ascending aorta compatible with aortoannular ectasia. Left ventricular enlargement can be demonstrated as well.

Cine-GE images can be used for quantitative evaluation of valvular regurgitation based on the area of the signal void corresponding to the regurgitant flow jet in diastole [33], better demonstrated on the coronal plane centered on the left ventricular outflow tract (Fig. 5.**10**) and the long axis of the left ventricle. Because the abnormal regurgitant flow jet is a three-dimensional structure and may change shape and direction from one patient to another it is preferable to assess the area of signal void on both planes.

The best way to quantify the degree of aortic regurgitation is to use VEC-MR. By using a plane perpendicular to the direction of flow on the ascending aorta at the level of the right pulmonary artery to avoid artifacts, eddy currents and complex motions of the valve, one can measure for each frame, the cross-sectional area (A) by tracing a region of interest (ROI) manually positioned around the aorta on the magnitude images. Then, this ROI is transferred from the magnitude image to the corresponding phase image for each frame, thus allowing through-plane measurement of the average velocity (AvV) (Fig. 5.**10**). The product of A and AvV in the ROI gives the instantaneous flow at each time frame. Integration of flow values for each frame estimates blood flow volumes [7]. Diastolic retrograde aortic flow equals aortic regurgitant volume. After plotting flow versus time during the cardiac cycle the area bounded by the curve under the baseline represents the regurgitant volume, allowing calculation of the regurgitant fraction [34] (Fig. 5.**5**).

5.3.3 Combined Aortic Stenosis and Regurgitation

Combined aortic stenosis and insufficiency is a condition encountered in the evolution of an abnormal bicuspid aortic valve. It is important to determine the dominant lesion, however in some cases the pathophysiology process may be balanced. A bicuspid aortic valve can be demonstrated by MR images as well but is less accurate than echocardiography. Cine-GE images can be used for quantitative evaluation of valvular stenosis and regurgitation as described above (Fig. 5.**11**). However, the best method for quantifying the degree of stenosis and regurgitation is the VEC-MR technique as described previously.

5.3.4 Mitral Stenosis

Mitral stenosis due to restricted opening of the mitral valve during diastole results in left ventricular inlet obstruction with a diastolic pressure gradient between the left atrium and the left ventricle. Rheumatic disease is the most common cause of mitral stenosis. Fusion of the commissures and thickening of the leaflets are affected but chordae tendinae can be affected as well. Doppler echocardiography is the procedure of choice for evaluating the degree of mitral stenosis and is sufficient in the majority of cases to plan the therapeutic options. MRI can be useful in cases where the Doppler

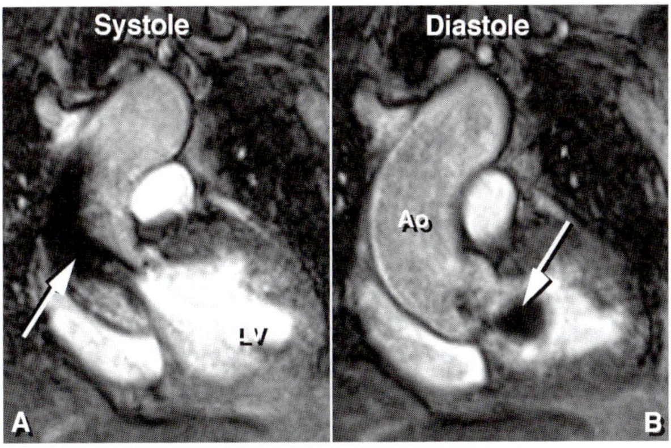

Fig. 5.**11** Coronal cine-GE images of a patient with a combined aortic stenosis and regurgitation due to long-standing bicuspid aortic valve. A large signal void is clearly visible in systole (arrow on **A**) related to the valve stenosis and a small signal void is demonstrated in diastole (arrow on **B**) related to mild aortic regurgitation.
Ao = aorta, LV = left ventricle.

study is inconsistent with clinical data or insufficient, particularly when the acoustic window is limited and in cases of complex flow patterns that are better demonstrated by MRI which displays the entire abnormal flow jet in any plane or direction. Conversely, MRI will be limited in cases of atrial fibrillation, very often encountered in mitral stenosis, where a potential source of error can occur in the measurements.

Spin-echo images may demonstrate thickening and bulging of the leaflets, dilatation of the left atrium whereas the left ventricle is small. Cine-GE images can be used to evaluate the degree of mitral stenosis based on the size and extent of the abnormal flow jet during diastole in the left ventricle and associated anatomic findings (valve leaflets thickening and bulging, reduced valve motion, left atrial enlargement). The optimal planes for identifying the signal void corresponding to the abnormal flow jet are the 4 chamber view and the coronal oblique plane encompassing the left atrium and the left ventricle. With the help of VEC-MR, the calculation of the maximum velocity (V_{max}) within the stenotic jet can performed either on planes perpendicular or parallel to the direction of flow. The pressure gradient across the stenotic mitral valve can be derived using the modified Bernoulli equation described previously [35] (Fig. 5.**12**).

5.3.5 Mitral Regurgitation

Mitral regurgitation can be due to abnormalities of mitral annulus, mitral leaflets, chordae tendinae and the papillary muscles. The most frequent causes are rheumatic disease where the cusps are scarred and fibrotic, endocarditis, where the cusps are destroyed, dysfunction due to infarction, dilated heart due to congestive heart failure, prolapse and congenital. The major hemodynamic consequence of mitral regurgitation is an increase of total stroke volume of the left ventricle. The need for surgery is determined by the severity of symptoms and if the ejection fraction falls towards 60% or left ventricular end-systolic dimension approaches 45 mm as determined by Doppler echocardiography [36]. However, more precise measurements of the degree of

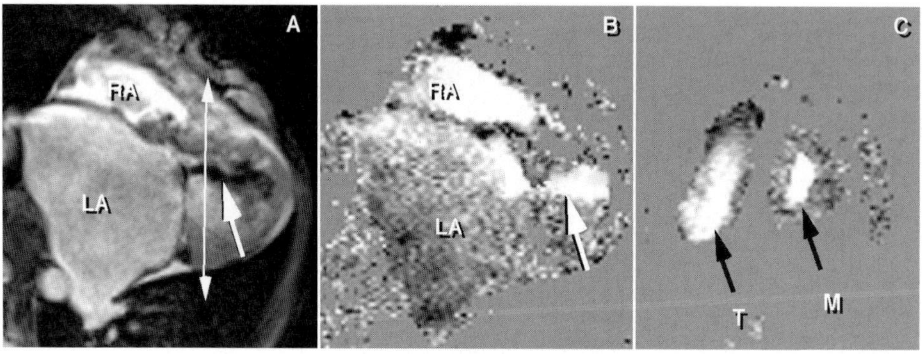

Fig. 5.**12** Four-chamber cine-GE image (**A**) and corresponding phase VEC-MR images (**B**, **C**) of a patient with a tight mitral stenosis. A massive enlargement of the left atrium (LA) and the abnormal flow jet due to mitral stenosis in diastole (arrow) are demonstrated on cine-GE images. Note the size and the extension of the jet reaching the apex of the left ventricle compatible with a severe stenosis. The calculation of the peak velocity (V_{max}) was performed by placing a ROI into the abnormal flow jet on the plane parallel to the direction of flow identical to the four-chamber view (arrow on **B**) (in-plane velocity measurement). This was done as well on a plane perpendicular to the direction of flow, just below the mitral valve (M on **C**) (through-plane velocity measurement) indicated by the double-headed arrow on **A**. The peak velocity was calculated to 2.3 m/sec which corresponds to a pressure gradient across the mitral valve of 22 mm Hg. T = tricuspid flow.

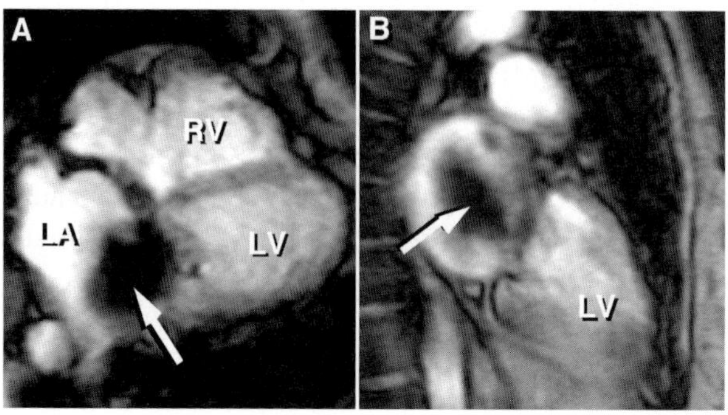

Fig. 5.**13** Cine-GE images in the 4 chamber view (**A**) and in the coronal oblique plane encompassing the left atrium (LA) and the left ventricle (LV) (**B**) show enlargement of the LA and the abnormal flow jet due to mitral regurgitation in systole (arrows). In this patient, evaluation of the severity of mitral regurgitation was accomplished by measuring the ventricular volumes on cine-GE images. The regurgitant fraction was equal to 0.50. RV = right ventricle.

regurgitation are also important. Measurements of the area and length of mitral regurgitant jet by Doppler echocardiography are semiquantitative. A direct quantitative non-invasive assessment of the regurgitant volume can be accurately performed by MRI [32].

On spin-echo images the left ventricle and the left atrium are enlarged. Cine-GE images can be used to evaluate the severity of mitral regurgitation based on the area of the signal void emanating from the insufficient mitral valve corresponding to the

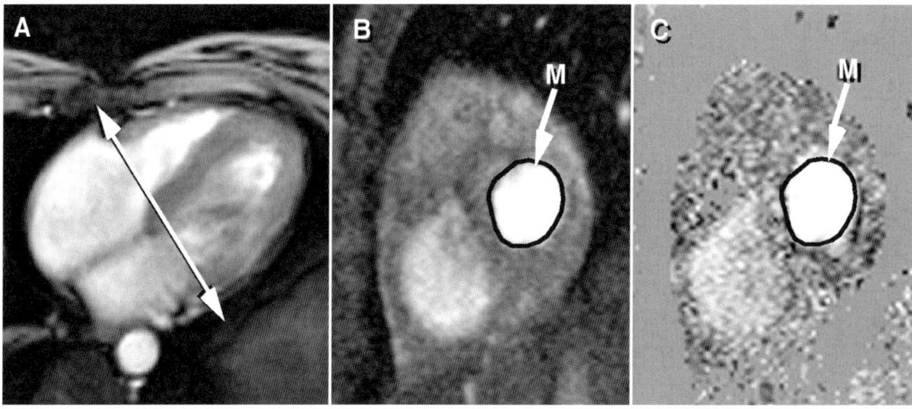

Fig. 5.**14** Cine-GE images in the 4 chamber view (**A**), and magnitude (**B**) and phase (**C**) VEC-MR images perpendicular to the mitral (M) and tricuspid annuli (indicated by the double headed arrow on **A**) in a patient with mitral regurgitation. This plane allows the calculation of mitral diastolic inflow that will be compared with aortic outflow which are identical in normal subjects. Left ventricular inflow is increased in mitral regurgitation.

regurgitant flow jet in systole. This flow void is better demonstrated on the four-chamber view and on the coronal oblique view encompassing the left atrium and left ventricle (Fig. 5.**13**). A good correlation has been found between the ratio of maximal flow void area to left atrial and left ventricular area and severity of mitral regurgitation estimated by pulsed and color Doppler [37,38]. As mentioned above it is preferable to assess the area of signal void on both planes. In spite of that, it could be difficult to choose the image on which the signal loss shows the larger size because the regurgitant jet may change shape and direction throughout the cardiac cycle.

A good method for evaluating the severity of a mitral regurgitation is to calculate the regurgitant fraction by measuring the ventricular volumes as described previously (Figs. 5.**2** and 5.**3**). However, as with cardiac scintigraphy this calculation is valid only for patients with a single regurgitant valve [7,10].

Mitral regurgitation can also be quantified by using VEC-MRI in comparing diastolic inflow across the mitral annulus and systolic outflow across the ascending aorta. These values are nearly identical in normal subjects. Left ventricular inflow is increased in mitral regurgitation. The difference between the areas of the two curves corresponds to the volume of mitral regurgitation (Figs. 5.**14** and 5.**15**). With this method, patients with moderate or severe mitral regurgitation could be discriminated from normal subjects and patients with mild regurgitation [10,39].

Another way to calculate the regurgitant volume is to use VEC-MR by measuring flow in the ascending aorta and pulmonary artery on a plane perpendicular to the vessel. Flow is the product of the mean velocity in the vessel and the area of the vessel on each time frame during the cardiac cycle. Integration of the flow for all images during systole provides a measurement of the systolic output flow. Thus, stroke vo-

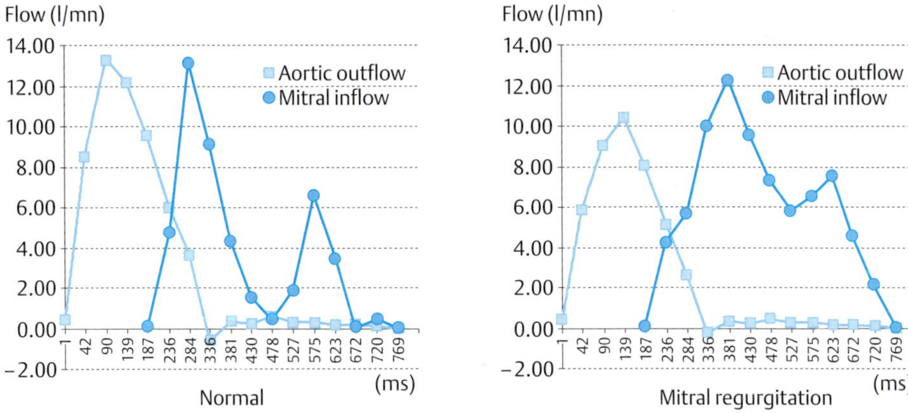

Fig. 5.**15** Graphs of mitral inflow and aortic outflow obtained on phase images performed perpendicular to the mitral annulus and perpendicular to the ascending aorta in a normal subject (left) and a patient with mitral regurgitation (right). These flows across mitral and aortic valves are nearly identical in normal subjects. Conversely, left ventricular inflow is increased in mitral regurgitation. The difference between the areas of the two curves corresponds to the volume of mitral regurgitation (left).

lumes of the left ventricle and the right ventricle can be calculated respectively. Regurgitant volume is the difference between the left ventricular stroke volume and the right ventricular stroke volume [10].

Probably the best way to quantify the volume of mitral regurgitation is to combine ventricular volume measurements by cine-GE sequences and calculation of forward flow in the aorta by VEC-MR. The left ventricular stroke volume index (LVSVI), which is the difference between left ventricular end-diastolic volume index (LVEDVI) and end-systolic volume index (LVESVI), will be calculated on cine-GE images as described above. The left ventricular cardiac index (LVCI) will be calculated as the product of LVSVI and heart rate. Then, the regurgitant volume index (RVI) will be calculated by subtracting the forward cardiac index (FCI) measured with VEC-MR on a plane perpendicular to the proximal aorta from LVCI. The regurgitant fraction will be determined by dividing RVI by LVCI. These measurements correlated well with those obtained by catheterization and angiography where the regurgitant flow is calculated by subtracting the forward cardiac output (measured by the Fick principle or indicator dilution) from the left ventricular output (measured by contrast ventriculography) [40].

5.3.6 Pulmonary Stenosis

Valvular pulmonary stenosis is usually a congenital anomaly due to fusion of the leaflets at the commissures which prevents them from opening completely during systole, and is often well tolerated over many years. In severe valvular pulmonary

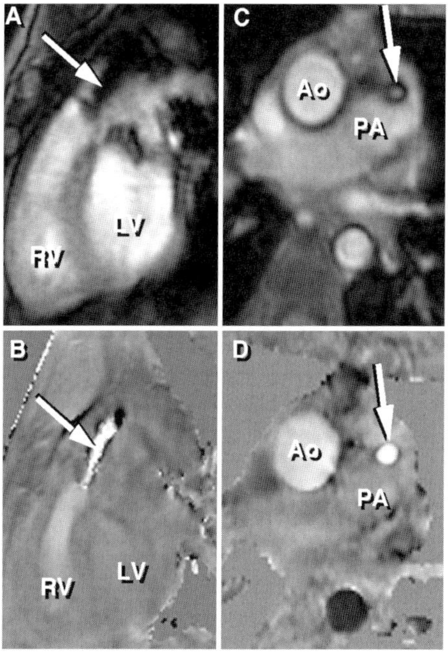

Fig. 5.**16** Cine-GE image (**A**) and corresponding VEC phase image (**B**) in the sagittal plane centered on the pulmonary trunk in a patient with pulmonary valve stenosis. The bulging of the pulmonary leaflets and the abnormal flow jet emanating from the stenotic valve in systole (arrow), responsible for poststenotic dilatation at the pulmonary bifurcation are demonstrated on **A**. Velocity was encoded vertically on **B** (in-plane velocity measurement), allowing calculation of the maximum velocity in the abnormal flow jet. Magnitude (**C**) and corresponding phase (**D**) acquired in a plane perpendicular to the pulmonary trunk (through-plane velocity measurement) allow the calculation of the valve area (arrow on **C**) as well as an additional measurement of the maximum velocity within the stenotic jet. In this case the maximum velocity was equal to 5 m/s corresponding to a gradient of 100 mm Hg.

stenosis, patients present with symptoms of chronic right ventricular failure. At present, one of the therapeutic modalities of pulmonary stenosis is percutaneous valvuloplasty. Doppler echocardiography is the procedure of choice in evaluating the degree of pulmonary stenosis and is sufficient in the majority of cases to plan the therapeutic options. MRI can be useful in cases where the Doppler study is inconsistent with clinical data or insufficient, particularly when the acoustic window is limited. MRI, which displays the entire abnormal flow jet in any plane or direction, can provide a direct measurement of the degree of stenosis. Spin-echo images can demonstrate bulging of pulmonary valve, right ventricular hypertrophy and poststenotic dilatation of the pulmonary artery at the level of the bifurcation [41].

Cine-GE images can be used to evaluate the severity of valvular stenosis based on the size and extent of the abnormal flow jet and associated findings (valve leaflets thickening and bulging, reduced valve motion, right ventricular enlargement and/or wall thickening) encountered in pulmonary stenotic valves. The optimal plane for identifying the signal void corresponding to the abnormal flow jet is the sagittal plane centered on the pulmonary trunk. It shows the bulging of the pulmonary valve leaflets and the abnormal jet emanating from the stenotic valve responsible for poststenotic dilatation at the bifurcation (jet lesion) (Fig. 5.**16**). With the help of VEC-MR, the calculation of the maximum velocity (V_{max}) within the stenotic jet can be carried out either on planes perpendicular or parallel to the direction of flow (Fig. 5.**16**). The pressure gradient across the stenotic valve can be derived using the modified Bernoulli equation.

5.3.7 Pulmonary Regurgitation

Pulmonary regurgitation can be caused by dilatation of the valve annulus secondary to pulmonary hypertension, endocarditis and complications of surgical treatment for pulmonary stenosis, tetralogy of Fallot or other cono-truncal malformations. This is particularly the case when reconstruction of the outflow tract does not include valvular apparatus. The major hemodynamic consequence of pulmonary regurgitation is an increase of end-diastolic volume of the right ventricle. Doppler echocardiography and angiography have limitations in evaluating right ventricular morphology and function. MRI with its multiplanar capability and the three-dimensional nature of the technique allows one to display right ventricular dilatation and hypertrophy more accurately than by echocardiography. Moreover, a direct measurement of regurgitant volume in the right ventricle as well as right ventricular function is also possible with MRI.

On spin-echo images the right ventricle, particularly the outflow tract, is usually dilated. Cine-GE images can be used to evaluate the severity of pulmonary regurgitation based on the area of signal void generated by the regurgitant jet in diastole. This regurgitant flow is best demonstrated on sagittal plane centered on the right ventricle outflow tract and pulmonary artery (Fig. 5.**17**).

The best method for quantifying the degree of pulmonary regurgitation is VEC-MRI [42]. By using a plane perpendicular to the direction of flow on the pulmonary trunk just below the bifurcation, one can measure for each frame, the cross-sectional area (A) of the pulmonary artery by tracing a region of interest (ROI) manually positioned around the pulmonary artery on the magnitude images. Then, this ROI is transferred

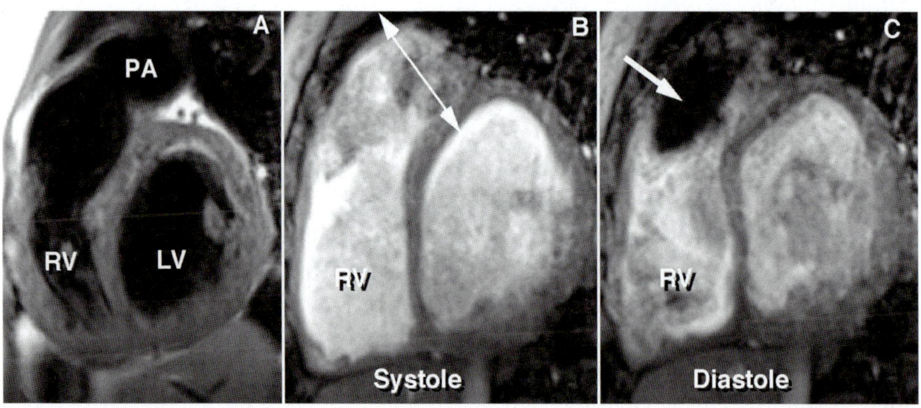

Fig. 5.**17** Spin-echo (**A**) and cine-GE images (**B**, **C**) in the sagittal plane centered on the pulmonary trunk (PA) and the outflow tract of the right ventricle (RV) of a patient with pulmonary regurgitation, operated for tetralogy of Fallot several years earlier. Note the large signal void in diastole (arrow on **C**) suggestive of severe pulmonary regurgitation as well as right ventricular enlargement and hypertrophy. Double-headed arrow shows the plane perpendicular to the pulmonary trunk used for through-plane calculation of pulmonary flow on the next image.

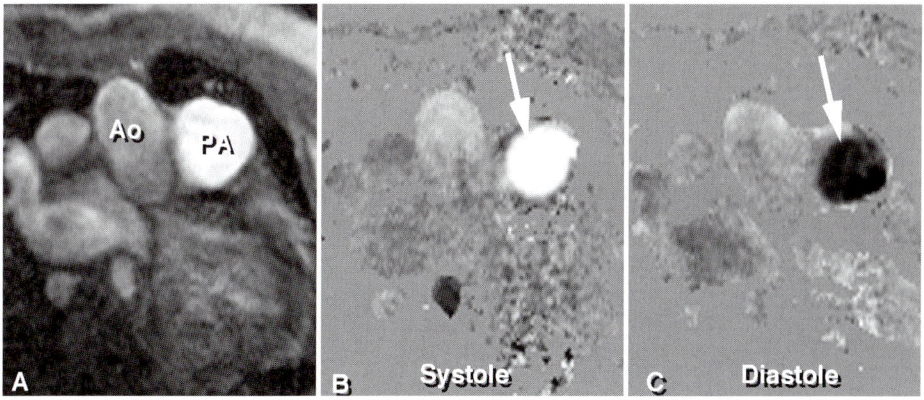

Fig. 5.**18** Magnitude (**A**) and phase (**B**, **C**) VEC-MR images of a patient operated for tetralogy of Fallot several years earlier with pulmonary regurgitation (same patient as in Fig. 5.**17**) acquired in a plane perpendicular to the pulmonary trunk (through-plane velocity measurement) in systole (**B**) and in diastole (**C**). Systolic image shows bright signal (arrow) in the pulmonary artery (PA) reflecting forward flow whereas diastolic image shows dark signal (arrow) in the PA reflecting flow in the opposite direction (i.e., pulmonary regurgitation).

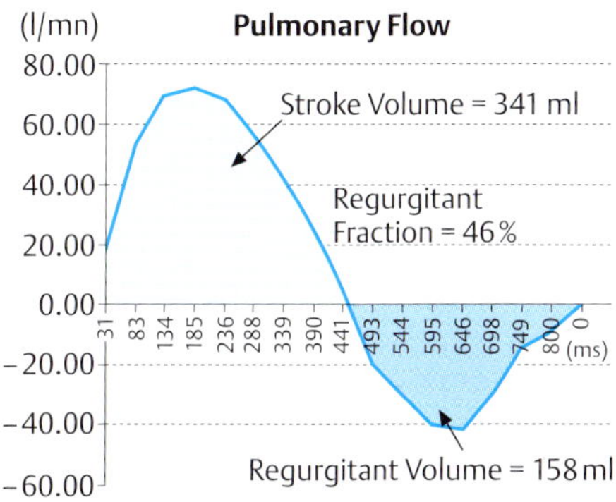

Fig. 5.**19** Graph of flow volume curve versus time in the pulmonary artery of the same patient as in Figs. 5.**17** and 5.**18** shows the stroke volume in systole (light blue) whereas the latter part of the curve (dark blue) below the baseline represents the retrograde flow in diastole. Regurgitant volume is calculated as the area bounded by the curve under the baseline during diastole. The regurgitant fraction, which is regurgitant volume divided by the stroke volume has been calculated as 46%, which indicates a severe pulmonary regurgitation.

from the magnitude image to the corresponding phase image for each frame, thus allowing measurement of the average velocity (AvV) (Fig. 5.**18**). The product of A and AvV in the ROI gives the instantaneous flow at each time frame. Integration of flow values for each frame estimates blood flow volumes. Diastolic retrograde aortic flow equals pulmonary regurgitant volume. After plotting flow versus time during the cardiac cycle the area bounded by the curve under the baseline represents the regurgitant volume, allowing calculation of the regurgitant fraction (Fig. 5.**19**).

5.3.8 Tricuspid Regurgitation

Tricuspid regurgitation can be due to endocarditis, rheumatic disease, dilatation of the right ventricle and the tricuspid annulus secondary to mitral valvulopathy or pulmonary hypertension, dysfunction due to infarction, trauma, carcinoid syndrome, Marfan syndrome and congenital (Ebstein's anomaly). The major hemodynamic consequence of tricuspid regurgitation is an increase of total stroke volume of the right ventricle.

On spin-echo images the right ventricle and the right atrium as well as vena cava and hepatic veins are enlarged. Cine-GE images can be used to evaluate tricuspid regurgitation based on the area of the signal void corresponding to the regurgitant flow jet in systole which is better demonstrated on the four chamber view and on the coronal oblique view encompassing the right atrium and the right ventricle (Fig. 5.**20**).

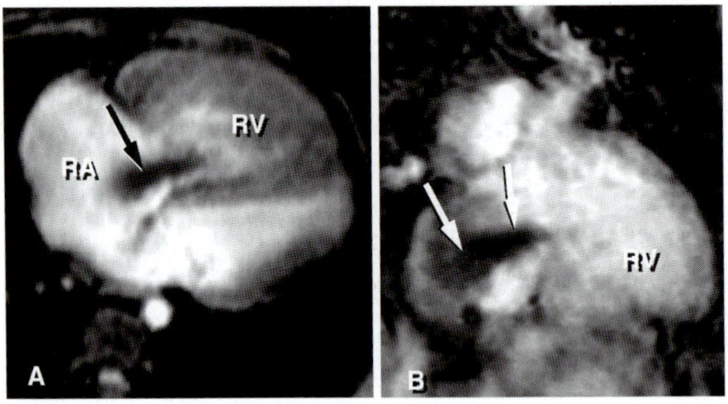

Fig. 5.**20** Cine-GE images in the four chamber view (**A**) and in the coronal oblique plane encompassing the right atrium (RA) and the right ventricle (RV) (**B**) show enlargement of the RA and the abnormal flow jet due to tricuspid regurgitation in systole (arrows). The large signal void, reaching the right atrial wall on the coronal plane is suggestive of severe tricuspid regurgitation.

As in Doppler echocardiography, VEC-MRI allows quantification of the regurgitation by measuring the maximum velocity (V_{max}) in the regurgitant tricuspid flow jet [43]. Furthermore, right ventricular systolic pressure (RVs·P) and pulmonary artery systolic pressure (PA·P) can be estimated from this measurement. The pressure difference between right ventricle and right atrium is calculated by using the modified Bernoulli equation: deduced from this maximum velocity by using the modified Bernoulli equation:

$$\Delta P = 4 \cdot (V_{max})^2 \qquad RVs \cdot P = Pa \cdot P = Ra \cdot P + \Delta P$$

where RA·P is the right atrial pressure estimated to 10 mm Hg.

5.3.9 Combined Mitral and Tricuspid Regurgitation

In cases of associated mitral and tricuspid insufficiencies, a cine-GE sequence in the four chamber view displays both regurgitant flow jets and the degree of regurgitation can be appreciated by the length and area of the flow void as described previously (Fig. 5.**21**). As mentioned before, the method based on the volume measurements cannot be applied in this case. VEC-MRI techniques described previously are the only methods capable of adequately quantifying the severity of both regurgitations.

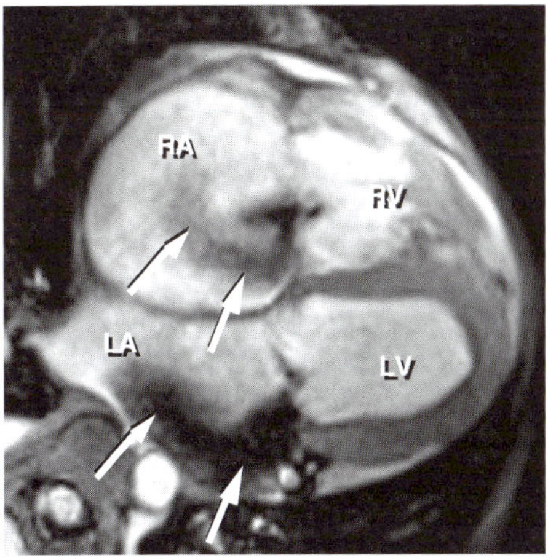

Fig. 5.**21** Combined mitral and tricuspid regurgitations in a four chamber cine-GE image. Enlargement of the right (RA) and the left (LA) atria, as well as large systolic regurgitant flow voids (arrows) are suggestive of severe mitral and tricuspid insufficiencies. For the quantification of the degree of regurgitation, the method based on the volume measurements cannot be applied in this case. RV= right ventricle, LV= left ventricle.

5.3.10 Prosthetic Valves and Endocarditis

Endocarditis is a severe complication after valvular replacement by a mechanical prosthesis and diagnosis must be made as quickly as possible because reoperation is usually mandatory. Transesophageal echocardiography is unique for the assessment of valvular morphology, especially in demonstrating vegetations in infective endocarditis. However, magnetic resonance imaging plays an important role in diagnosing

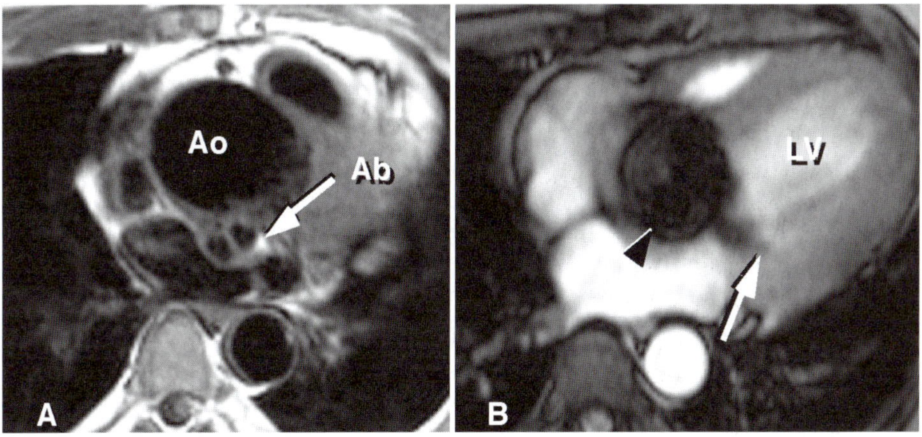

Fig. 5.**22** Spin-echo (**A**) and cine-GE images (**B**) of a patient with rheumatic disease previously operated with a St Jude aortic prosthetic valve who presented with fever. A paravalvular abscess (Ab) situated behind the aortic annulus and prolapsing into the left atrium is well demonstrated. Note on the cine-GE image the artifact due to the prosthesis (arrow-head) and a small signal void extending from the prosthetic valve into the left ventricle (LV) in diastole, corresponding to a mild aortic regurgitation (arrow).

paravalvular abscesses associated with infectious processes which are always difficult to demonstrate by echocardiography because of the artifacts due to the prosthesis, even with a transesophageal technique. Patients with current prosthetic valves can be imaged safely in high field magnets [32]. Spin-echo images can demonstrate the exact location of the abscess and connections with cavities and great vessels. Cine-GE images, even with the artifact created by the prosthesis, are unique to evaluate the repercussions on the function of the valve and connections of the abscess with the right and left cavities or great vessels and VEC-MR permits the quantification of associated regurgitation (Fig. 5.**22**).

5.4 References

1. Bolger A, Eigler N, Maurer G. Quantifying valvular regurgitation: Limitations and inherent assumptions of Doppler techniques. Circulation 1988; 78: 1316–1318.
2. Simpson I, Sahn D. Quantification of valvular regurgitation by Doppler echocardiography. Circulation 1991; 84 (suppl I): 188–192.
3. Carabello BA, Crawford FA. Valvular heart disease. N Engl J Med 1997; 307: 1362–1367.
4. Currie PJ, Seward JB, Reeder GS, et al. Continuous wave Doppler echocardiographic assessment of the severity of calcific aortic stenosis: A simultaneous Doppler-catheter correlative study in 100 adult patients. Circulation 1985; 71: 1162–1169.
5. Cheitlin M. Valvular heart disease. Management and intervention. Circulation 1991; 84 (suppl I): 259–264.
6. Globits S, Higgins CB. Assessment of valvular heart disease by magnetic resonance imaging. Am Heart J 1995; 129: 369–381.
7. Duerinckx AJ, Higgins CB. Valvular heart disease. Radiol Clin North Am 1994; 32: 613–630.
8. Didier D, Ratib O, Lerch R, Friedli B. Detection and quantification of valvular heart disease with dynamic cardiac MR imaging. RadioGraphics 2000; 20: 1279–1299.
9. Sondergaard L, Stahlberg F, Thomsen C. Magnetic resonance imaging of valvular heart disease. J Magn Reson Imaging 1999; 10: 627–638.
10. Higgins CB, Sakuma H. Heart disease: Functional evaluation with MR imaging. Radiology 1996; 199: 307–315.
11. Mostbeck GH, Caputo GR, Higgins CB. MR measurements of blood flow in the cardiovascular system. AJR 1992; 159: 453–461.
12. Rebergen SA, van der Wall EE, Doornbos J, et al. Magnetic resonance measurements of velocity and flow: Technique, validation and cardiovascular applications. Am Heart J 1993; 126: 1439–1456.
13. Ratib O, Didier D, Chatelain P, Righetti A, Lerch R, Townsend D. Standard views in cardiac multimodality tomographic imaging. Am J Card Imaging 1995; 9: 67–76.
14. Didier D, Ratib O, Friedli B, et al. Cine gradient-echo MR imaging in the evaluation of cardiovascular diseases. RadioGraphics 1993; 13: 561–573.

15. Suzuki JI, Caputo GR, Kondo C, Higgins CB. Cine MR imaging of valvular heart disease: display and imaging parameters affect the size of the signal void caused by valvular regurgitation. AJR 1990; 155: 723–727.
16. Baldy C, Doueck P, Croisille P, et al. Automated myocardial edge detection from breath-hold cine-MR images: Evaluation of left ventricular volumes and mass. Magn Reson Imaging 1994; 12: 589–592.
17. Nayler GL, Firmin DN, Longmore DB. Blood flow imaging by cine magnetic resonance. J Comput Assist Tomogr 1986; 10: 715–722.
18. Bogren HG, Buonocore MH. Blood flow measurements in the aorta and major arteries with MR velocity mapping. JMRI 1994; 4: 119–130.
19. Higgins CB, Caputo G, Wendland MF, Saeed M. Measurement of blood flow and perfusion in the cardiovascular system. Invest Radiol 1992; 27: S66–S71.
20. Mohiaddin RH, Pennell DJ. MR blood flow measurement. Clinical application in the heart and circulation. Cardiol Clin 1998; 16: 161–187.
21. Firmin DN, Nayler GL, Kilner PJ, et al. The applications of phase shifts in NMR for flow measurements. Magn Reson Med 1990; 14: 230–241.
22. Kondo C, Caputo GR, Semelka R, et al. Right and left ventricular stroke volume measurements with velocity encoded cine NMR imaging: in vitro and in vivo evaluation. AJR 1991; 157: 9–16.
23. Utz JA, Herfkens RJ, Heinsimer JA, Shimakawa A, Glover G, Pelc N. Valvular regurgitation: Dynamic MR imaging. Radiology 1988; 168: 91–94.
24. Nishimura T, Yamada N, Itoh A, Miyatake K. Cine MR imaging in mitral regurgitation: comparison with color Doppler flow imaging. AJR 1989; 153: 721–724.
25. Wagner S, Aufferman W, Buser P, et al. Diagnostic accuracy and estimation of the severity of valvular regurgitation from the signal void on cine magnetic resonance images. Am Heart J 1989; 118: 760–767.
26. Sechtem U, Pflugfelder PW, Cassidy MM, et al. Mitral or aortic regurgitation: quantification of regurgitant volumes with cine MR imaging. Radiology 1988; 167: 425–430.
27. Honda N, Machida K, Hashimoto M, et al. Aortic regurgitation: quantitation with MR imaging velocity mapping. Radiology 1993; 186: 189–194.
28. Szolar DH, Sakuma H, Higgins CB. Cardiovascular applications of magnetic resonance flow and velocity measurements. JMRI 1996; 1: 78–89.
29. Sechtem U, Pflugfelder PW, White RD, et al: Cine MR imaging: Potential for the evaluation of cardiovascular function. AJR 1987; 148: 239–246.
30. Sondergaard L, Hildebrandt P, Lindvig K, et al. Valve area and cardiac output in aortic stenosis. Am Heart J 1993; 127: 1156–1164.
31. Kilner PJ, Manzara CC, Mohiaddin RH, et al. Magnetic resonance jet velocity mapping in mitral and aortic valve stenosis. Circulation 1993; 87: 1239–1248.
32. Wyttenbach R, Bremerich J, Saeed M, Higgins CB. Integrated MR imaging approach to valvular heart disease. Cardiol Clin 1998; 16: 277–294.

33. Pflugfelder PW, Landzberg JS, Cassidy MM, et al. Comparison of cine MR imaging with Doppler echocardiography for the evaluation of aortic regurgitation. AJR 1989; 152: 729–735.
34. Dulce MC, Mostbeck GH, O'Sullivan M, Cheitlin M, Caputo GR, Higgins CB. Severity of aortic regurgitation. Interstudy reproducibility of measurements with velocity-encoded cine MR imaging. Radiology 1992; 185: 235–240.
35. Heidenreich PA, Steffens J, Fujita N, et al. Evaluation of mitral stenosis with velocity-encoded cine-magnetic resonance imaging. Am J Cardiol 1995; 75: 365–369.
36. Carabello BA, Crawford FA: Valvular heart disease. N Engl J Med 1997; 307: 1362–1367.
37. Aurigemma G, Reichek N, Schiebler M, Axel L. Evaluation of mitral regurgitation by cine magnetic resonance imaging. Am J Cardiol 1990; 66: 621–625.
38. Nishimura T, Yamada N, Itoh A, Miyatake K. Cine MR imaging in mitral regurgitation: Comparison with color Doppler flow imaging. AJR 1989; 153:721–724.
39. Fujita N, Chazouilleres AF, Hartiala JJ, et al. Quantification of mitral regurgitation by velocity-encoded cine magnetic resonance imaging. J Am Coll Cardiol 1994; 23: 951–958.
40. Hundley WG, Li HF, Willard JE, et al. Magnetic resonance imaging assessment of the severity of mitral regurgitation. Comparison with invasive techniques. Circulation 1995; 92: 1151–1158.
41. Didier D, Higgins CB, Fisher MR, et al. Gated magnetic resonance imaging in congenital heart disease: experience in initial 72 patients. Radiology 1986; 158: 227–235.
42. Rebergen SA, Niezen RA, Helbing WA, van der Wall EE, de Roos A. Cine gradient echo MR imaging and MR velocity mapping in the evaluation of congenital heart disease. RadioGraphics 1996; 16: 467–481.
43. Kayser HV, Stoel BC, van der Wall EE, van der Geest, de Roos A. MR velocity mapping of tricuspid flow: correction for through-plane motion. J Magn Reson Imaging 1997;7: 669–673.

6 Pericardial Disease and Cardiomyopathy

MR imaging is becoming the non-invasive method of choice for evaluating some pericardial and myocardial diseases as a complementary modality to echocardiography because it provides three-dimensional, anatomic and functional data with highly reproducible measurements. With the combinations of different imaging techniques such as spin-echo and/or fast spin-echo, cine gradient-echo and flow-sensitive imaging, MRI allows discrimination between these diseases by providing a better visualization of morphology, functional abnormalities and flow velocity throughout the cardiovascular structures.

This chapter reviews existing MR imaging techniques used to evaluate pericardial and myocardial diseases and discusses the diagnostic information that can be provided by these techniques. For dynamic examples of cine sequences of pericardial diseases and cardiomyopathy, see the fifth section in the CD-ROM.

6.1 Pericardial Diseases

6.1.1 Normal Pericardium

Pericardium, consisting of two thin layers of fibrous tissue lubricated by pericardial fluid appears on T1-weighted spin-echo images as a low signal intensity curved line surrounded by high signal intensity of the epicardial and mediastinal fat pads (Fig. 6.**1**). The pericardial cavity may contain up to 60 ml of serous fluid. The pericardial thickness as visualized by MRI, comprising the pericardial fluid is 1 to 3 mm [1,2]. The pericardial sinus and recesses are also readily demonstrated on MR images (Fig. 6.**1**) [3].

6.1.2 Pericardial Effusion and Inflammatory Pericarditis

Pericarditis may result from different etiologies including bacterial or viral infection, uremia, post-myocardial infarction, cardiac surgery, neoplasm, trauma and idiopathic. Tuberculous pericarditis is at present a rare cause of acute pericarditis except in immunosuppressed patients. Echocardiography is the initial procedure of choice for evaluating acute pericarditis. But echocardiography does not provide accurate assessment of pericardial thickness. In cases of persisting symptoms, MRI is a very effective technique because it displays the entire pericardium and pericardial space and the pericardial thickness can be easily assessed. On T1-weighted spin-echo images, the presence of pericardial thickening of the visceral and parietal layers associated with

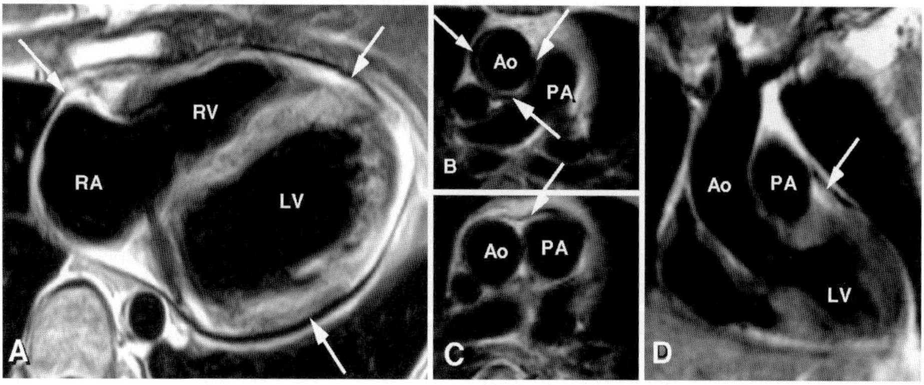

Fig. 6.**1** Normal pericardium.
On T1-weighted spin-echo images, pericardium appears as a thin dark line situated between the high signal intensity of the epicardial and mediastinal fat pads (arrows on **A**). Superior pericardial recesses are also readily shown on transverse (**B**, **C**) and coronal (**D**) images (arrows).
RA = right atrium, RV = right ventricle, LV = left ventricle, Ao = aorta, PA = pulmonary artery.

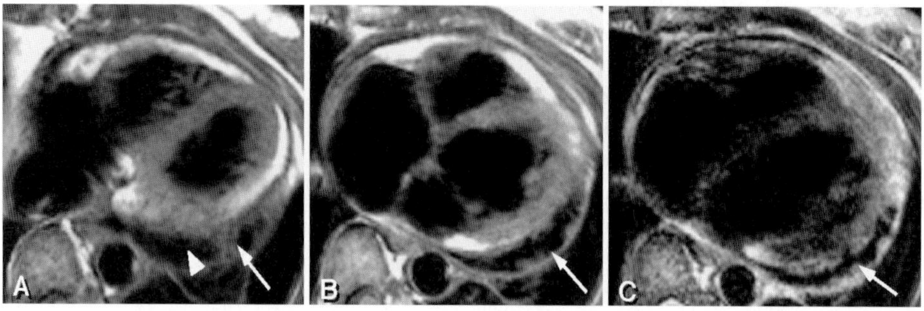

Fig. 6.**2** Inflammatory pericarditis.
T1-weighted (**A**, **B**) spin-echo images show thickening of the visceral and parietal pericardium associated with adhesions between the two layers (arrows). Associated pericardial effusion has low signal intensity (arrowhead). High signal intensity of the pericardial layers on the T2-weighted image (**C**) reinforces the diagnosis of acute or subacute inflammatory alterations (arrow).

adhesions between the two layers may be observed in the presence of intense inflammation. But it can be encountered in any inflammatory process and is not specific of a particular pericardial disease [1,4]. High signal intensity of the pericardial layers on T2-weighted images reinforces the diagnosis of acute or subacute inflammatory alterations. Associated pericardial effusion has low signal intensity on T1-weighted spin-echo images (Fig. 6.**2**). Cine MRI provides excellent evaluation of cardiac function and allows demonstration of the absence of evolution towards constrictive pericarditis. On cine MR images the pericardial effusion has high signal intensity, indicative of fluid motion within the pericardial sac.

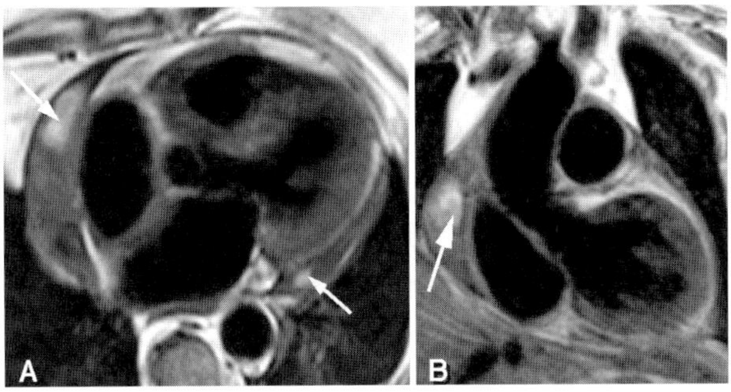

Fig. 6.**3** Hemorrhagic pericardial effusion.
On T1-weighted transverse (**A**) and coronal (**B**) spin-echo images hemorrhagic effusion is recognized as heterogeneous effusion containing areas of both medium and high signal intensity (arrows) due to the high signal of paramagnetic blood products and the variable age and nature of the blood.

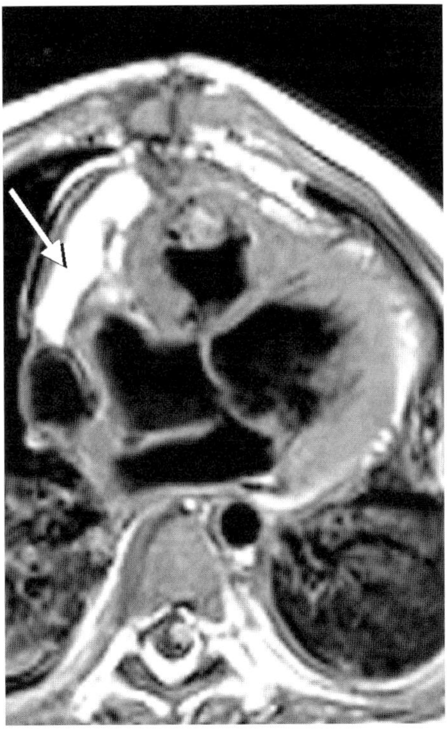

Fig. 6.**4** Postoperative pericardial hematoma. High signal intensity fluid within the pericardial sac identical to subcutaneous fat on T1-weighted spin-echo image (arrow) is characteristic for hematoma.

MRI is superior to echocardiography in defining the nature of pericardial effusion. Hemorrhagic effusion can be recognized on T1-weighted spin-echo images as heterogeneous effusion containing areas of both medium and high signal intensity due to the high signal of paramagnetic blood products and the variable age and nature of the blood. Clot and serum have different signal intensities that may vary over time [5] (Fig. 6.**3**). Postoperative pericardial hematoma can also be readily diagnosed on T1-weighted spin-echo images as high signal intensity fluid within the pericardial sac identical to subcutaneous fat [4] (Fig. 6.**4**).

6.1.3 Pericardial Thickening

Pericardium can be considered as thickened when its thickness is ≥4 mm. This thickening may result from infiltration of pericardial layers by inflammatory, fibrous or neoplastic tissue. It is often associated with pericardial constriction in symptomatic patients but may exist without constriction, particularly in postoperative patients for weeks after cardiac surgery [4]. Thickening appears as a low and/or medium intensity pericardial line depending on the associated effusion and calcification (Figs. 6.**5** and 6.**6**).

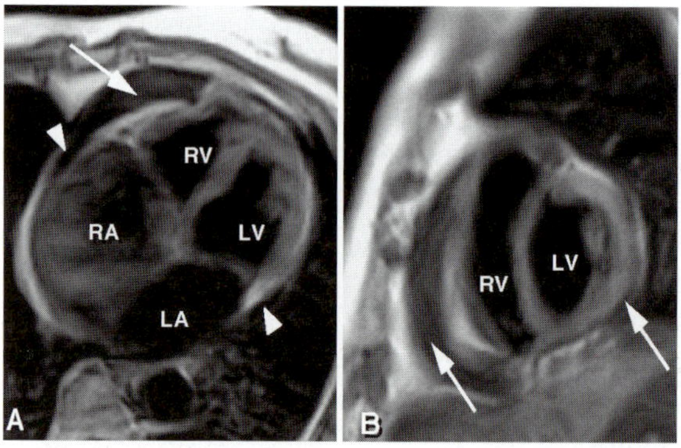

Fig. 6.**5** Constrictive pericarditis. T1 weighted transverse (**A**) and sagittal (**B**) spin-echo images show diffuse thickening (≥ 4 mm) of the pericardium predominantly over the right ventricle (RV) (arrows). Areas of low signal intensity represent pericardial calcifications and fluid collection between the two layers (arrow-heads). Right and left (LV) ventricles are small and tubular-shaped and the ventricular septum is sigmoid shaped. Right atrial (RA) enlargement is also demonstrated with substantial signal in the cavity consistent with stasis of blood. At surgery, extensive calcifications of the pericardium and viscous fluid collection were consistent with tuberculous constrictive pericarditis.
LA = left atrium.

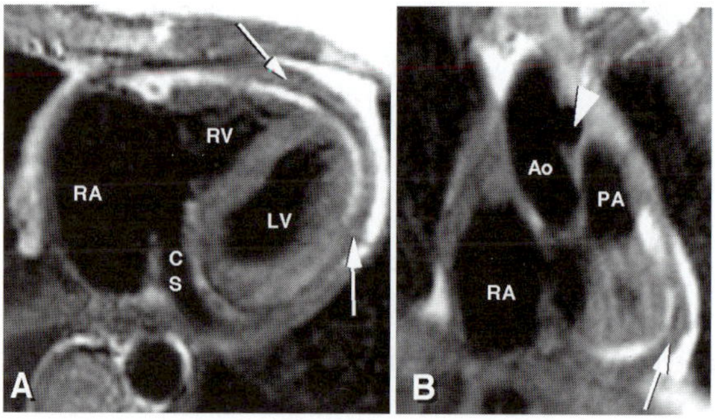

Fig. 6.**6** Post-traumatic constrictive pericarditis.
T1 weighted transverse (**A**) and coronal (**B**) spin-echo images show medium signal intensity diffuse thickening (> 4 mm) of the entire pericardium (arrows). Right and left ventricles (RV, LV) are small and tubular-shaped and the ventricular septum is sigmoid shaped. Right atrial (RA) and coronary sinus (CS) enlargements are demonstrated as well. A false aneurysm (arrow-head) is demonstrated on the left lateral border of the ascending aorta (Ao).
PA = pulmonary artery.

6.1.4 Constrictive Pericarditis

Constrictive pericarditis is characterized by fibrous scarring and thickening of the two layers of the pericardium secondary to an initial pericardial inflammation and is responsible for impairment of diastolic filling of the heart whereas systolic function is preserved. Tuberculosis was the main etiology of pericardial constriction before antibiotic therapy but at present 42% of the cases are of unknown etiology or idiopathic. Other etiologies are cardiac surgery, previous viral or bacterial infection, prior mediastinal irradiation, chronic renal failure, trauma, neoplastic infiltration, collagen diseases and post-myocardial infarction. Right heart failure is the usual clinical presentation. On chest X-rays, pericardial calcifications may be present but their absence does not exclude the disorder and some patients with pericardial calcifications do not have clinical manifestations of constriction [6,7]. The major clinical challenge is to distinguish constrictive pericarditis (treated surgically) from restrictive cardiomyopathy (treated medically). The clinical presentation may be similar as well as the hemodynamic profiles at cardiac catheterization with the classical "dip and plateau" or "square root" pattern on the diastolic tracing reflecting impaired ventricular filling during diastole. 2D and Doppler echocardiography provide criteria for distinguishing the two conditions. Prominent early diastolic filling, sudden displacement of the ventricular septum during early diastole, flattening of the mid and late diastolic motion of the left ventricular wall, premature opening of the pulmonary valve, variations in ventricular filling during the respiratory cycle favor constrictive pericarditis [6,8]. But echocardiography does not provide an accurate assessment of pericardial thickness. Both CT (with the ability to detect pericardial calcification as well) and MR are very effective to demonstrate pericardial thickening with a thickness of 4 mm or greater on spin-echo images. But this can be observed in the absence of constrictive pericarditis, particularly after cardiac surgery. Other MR findings are a dilatation of the inferior vena cava, coronary sinus and right atrium, an elongated tubular-shaped right ventricle and a sigmoid shaped ventricular septum [9,10] (Figs. 6.**5** and 6.**6**). Cine gradient-echo images in the four chamber and short axis planes provide additional information such as the typical abnormal motion (shivering) of the ventricular septum. There is a sudden anterior displacement of the ventricular septum during early diastole then the septum moves posteriorly and again anteriorly at end-diastole during atrial systole like a sail shivering in the wind (Figs. 6.**7** to 6.**9**). But this abnormal motion may be also encountered, although less frequently, in restrictive cardiomyopathy. The ventricular diastolic filling patterns help to distinguish both diseases as well. Rapid early diastolic filling is consistent with constriction whereas uniformly hindered filling is consistent with restriction. The signs demonstrated by spin-echo and cine-GE MR images allowing the differentiation between constrictive pericarditis and restrictive cardiomyopathy are summarized in Table 6.**1**.

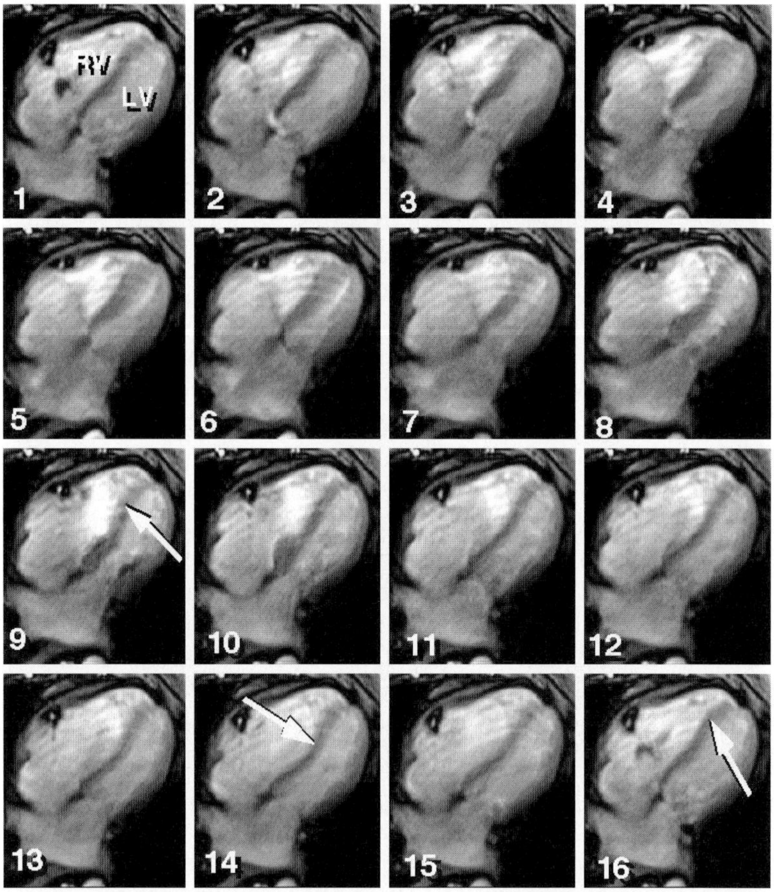

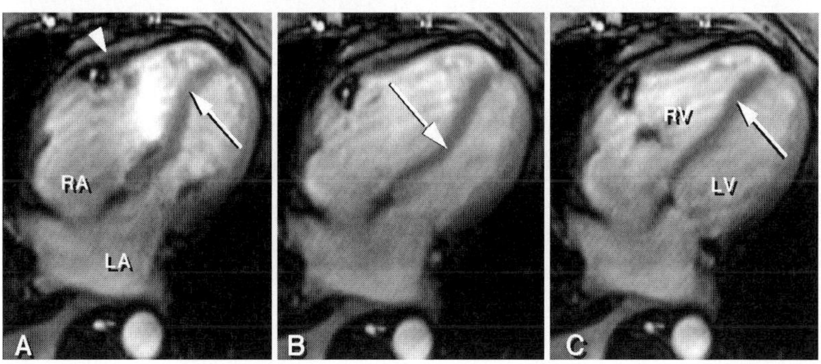

Figs. 6.**7** and 6.**8** Cine gradient-echo images in the four chamber plane in a patient with constrictive pericarditis.
Sixteen frames in an R-R interval (Fig. 6.**7**) and focus on diastolic frames (Fig. 6.**8**) show the two thickened layers (arrow-head), atrial enlargement, the tubular-shaped right (RV) and left (LV) ventricles as well as the typical abnormal motion (shivering) of the interventricular septum. There is a sudden anterior displacement of the interventricular septum during early diastole (arrow on A; frame 9), then the septum moves posteriorly (arrow on B; frame 14) and again anteriorly at end-diastole during atrial systole (arrow on C; frame 16) like a sail shivering in the wind.

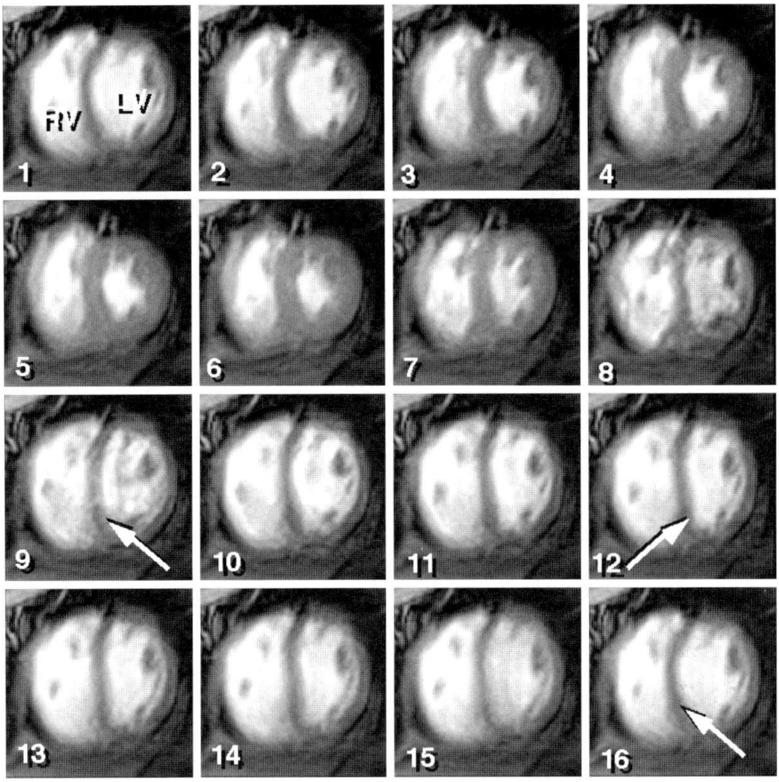

Fig. 6.**9**. Sixteen cine gradient-echo images in the short axis plane in a patient with constrictive pericarditis (same patient as Figs. 6.**7** and 6.**8**). The typical abnormal motion (shivering) of the interventricular septum is also well demonstrated (arrows).

Table 6.**1** Differentiation between constrictive pericarditis (CP) and restrictive cardiomyopathy (RC)

	CP	RC
Atrial, vena cava and coronary sinus enlargement	+	+
Abnormal morphology of ventricular cavities	tubular-shape RV	small ventricles
Tricuspid and/or mitral regurgitations	–	++
Decrease excursion of LV postero-lateral wall	+	+
Abnormal septal motion		
– paradoxical	+/–	+
– shivering	++	+/–
Septal systolic flattening	+	+
Pericardial thickening	++	–
Ventricular filling patterns	early filling	uniformly hindered filling

6.1.5 Pericardial Masses

MRI is very effective for demonstrating the location and nature of pericardial masses [11]. A pericardial cyst is usually located in the right or the left cardiophrenic angle and has low to medium signal intensity on T1-weighted spin-echo images depending on the protein concentration in the cyst (Fig. 6.**10**) and homogeneous high signal intensity on T2-weighted images. Among the other benign tumors, some have characteristic signs such as pericardial lipoma with high signal intensity identical to the subcutaneous fat on T1-weighted spin-echo images (Fig. 6.**11**).

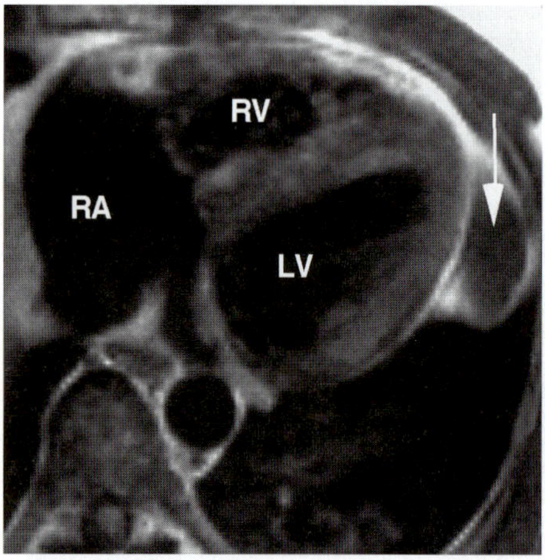

Fig. 6.**10** Pericardial cyst located in the left cardiophrenic angle (arrow).
The mass has low to medium signal intensity on T1-weighted spin-echo images and homogeneous high signal intensity on T2-weighted images (not shown).

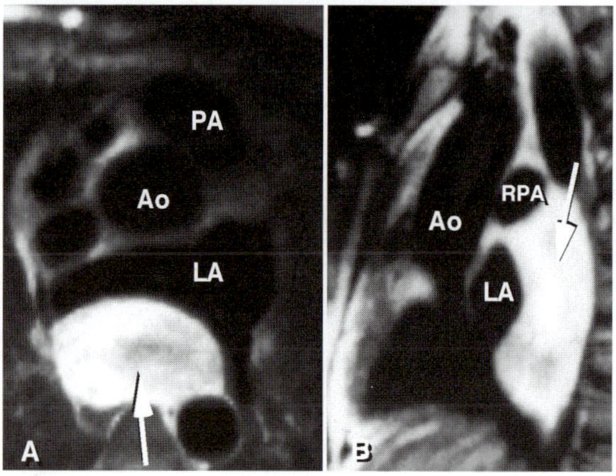

Fig. 6.**11** Pericardial lipoma situated within the oblique sinus of the pericardium.
High signal intensity mass identical to the signal of subcutaneous fat is shown behind the left atrium (LA) on transverse (**A**) and sagittal (**B**) T1-weighted spin-echo images.

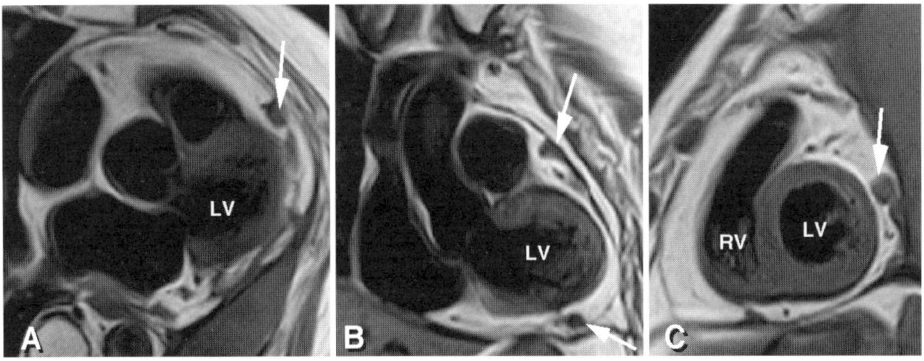

Fig. 6.**12** Pericardial metastases in a patient with bronchogenic carcinoma.
Transverse (**A**), coronal (**B**) and sagittal (**C**) T1-weighted spin-echo images show an enlargement of the pericardial line and the presence of multiple medium signal intensity masses within the pericardial space (arrows).
RV = right ventricle, LV = left ventricle.

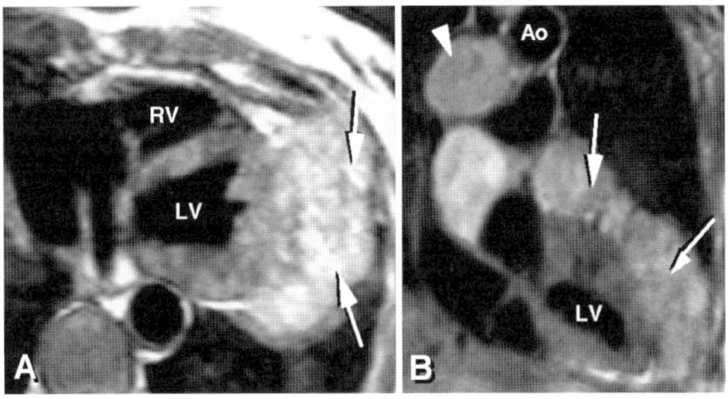

Fig. 6.**13** Pericardial metastases in a patient with previous melanoma. Direct invasion of the pericardium is demonstrated on transverse (**A**) and coronal (**B**) T1-weighted spin-echo images (arrows). Areas of high signal intensity are also shown, corresponding to associated hemorrhagic effusion. Metastases have reached the superior pericardial recesses as well (arrow-head). RV = right ventricle, LV = left ventricle, Ao = aorta.

Pericardial tumors are more frequently secondary to a bronchogenic carcinoma, melanoma or lymphoma. Primary malignant tumors are less frequent. Extension to the pericardium is recognized by obliteration or enlargement of the pericardial line (Fig. 6.12) associated or not with a pericardial effusion. In cases of hemorrhagic effusion associated with pericardial invasion, areas of high signal intensity can be demonstrated (Fig. 6.**13**). In almost all the pericardial tumors the signal reinforced after gadolinium injection. The most frequent pericardial masses are summarized in the Table 6.**2**.

Table 6.2 Pericardial masses

Primary tumors Benign	Malignant
Pericardial cyst	Mesothelioma
Teratoma	Sarcomas
Fibroma	
Lipoma	
Angioma	
Leiomyoma	
Pheochromocytoma	
Thymoma	
Hydatid cyst	
Secondary tumors	
Bronchogenic carcinoma	
Breast carcinoma	
Melanoma	
Lymphomas	
Leukemias	
Esophageal carcinoma	

6.2 Cardiomyopathies

6.2.1 Restrictive Cardiomyopathy

Restrictive cardiomyopathy is defined as heart-muscle disease that results in impaired ventricular filling in diastole due to a non-compliant ventricle whereas systolic function remains normal, at least early in the disease. It may affect either one or both ventricles and it is the least common of the cardiomyopathic disorders. The underlying pathologic process may be myocardial fibrosis or hypertrophy, or infiltration of the myocardium by abnormal substances [12]. The major causes of restrictive cardiomyopathy are as follows [13]:

1. Myocardial: non-infiltrative: idiopathic cardiomyopathy; infiltrative: amyloidosis, sarcoidosis, Gaucher's disease; storage diseases: hemochromatosis, glycogen storage disease.
2. Endomyocardial: endomyocardial fibrosis, hypereosinophilic (Löffler) syndrome, irradiation.

The major clinical challenge is to distinguish restrictive cardiomyopathy (usually treated medically) from constrictive pericarditis (treated surgically) as mentioned above. The clinical presentation may be similar as well as the hemodynamic profiles at cardiac catheterization reflecting impaired ventricular filling during diastole. Regurgitant murmur is common in restrictive cardiomyopathy whereas it is uncommon in constrictive pericarditis [14]. 2D and Doppler echocardiography provide criteria for distinguishing the two conditions. The presence of mitral or tricuspid regurgitation, increased early diastolic filling velocity (E wave ≥ 1.0 m/s), decreased atrial filling velocity (A wave ≤0.5 m/s), increased E/A ratio (≥ 2.0), decreased E wave deceleration time (≤ 150 ms), decreased isovolumetric relaxation time (≤70 ms) and minimal variations in ventricular filling during the respiratory cycle favor restrictive cardiomyopathy [15,16]. But echocardiography does not provide accurate assessment of pericardial thickness. Some findings summarized in Table 6.**1** help to differentiate both diseases. Both CT and MR are very effective to demonstrate pericardial thickening almost always absent in restrictive cardiomyopathy on spin-echo images (pericardial thickness ≤4 mm) [10]. Other MR findings include possible modification of the signal intensity ratio between myocardium and skeletal muscle (decreased in amyloidosis, idiopathic cardiomyopathy and hemochromatosis; increased in sarcoidosis) and thickening of the myocardium (amyloidosis) [16]. Cine gradient-echo images in the four chamber and short axis planes provide additional information such as tricuspid or mitral flow void corresponding to atrioventricular valve regurgitation and abnormal ventricular diastolic filling pattern. Rapid early diastolic filling is consistent with constriction whereas uniformly hindered filling is consistent with restriction (Figs.6.**14** and 6.**15**). Velocity-encoded cine MR sequences perpendicular to the atrioventricular annuli may demonstrate the same findings as Doppler echocardiography (Fig. 6.**16**). The ventricular filling curves obtained are similar to the Doppler curves and show the same modifications of the A and E waves (Fig. 6.**17**). Endomyocardial biopsy may reveal the specific cause of the restrictive cardiomyopathy [16].

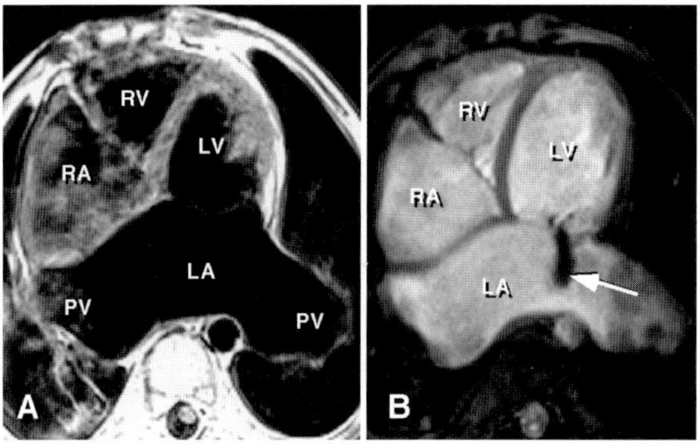

Fig. 6.**14** Restrictive cardiomyopathy.
T1-weighted spin-echo image (**A**) shows a massive enlargement of the right atrium (RA), the left (LA) atrium and the pulmonary veins (PV). Left (LV) and right (RV) ventricles are small and the presence of signal in the RA cavity is consistent with stasis of blood. Cine gradient-echo image (TE = 12) in the four chamber view (**B**) confirms these findings and demonstrate a flow void within the LA corresponding to mitral regurgitation (arrow).

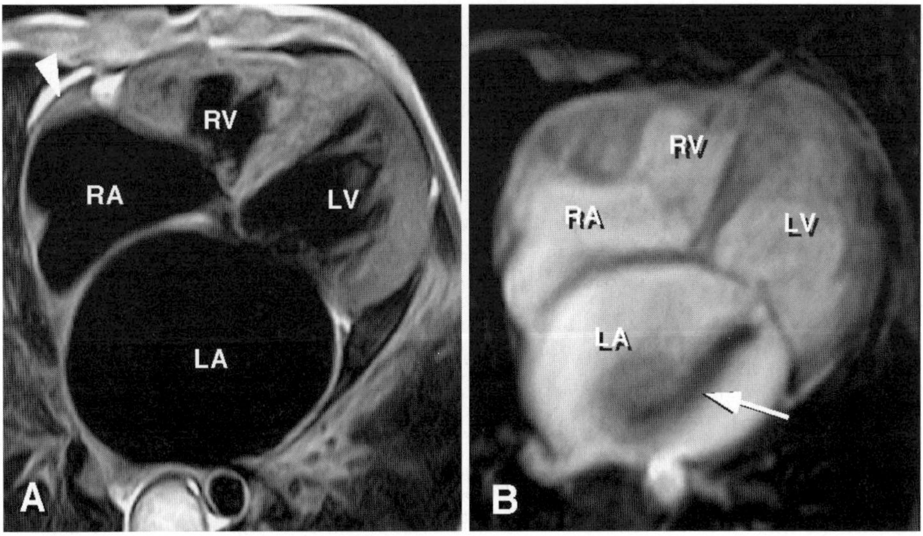

Fig. 6.**15** Restrictive cardiomyopathy.
T1-weighted spin-echo image (**A**) shows markedly dilated left atrium (LA) with atrial septum bulging towards the right atrium (RA) and normal size of the right (RV) and left (LV) ventricles. The pericardium is not thickened (≤ 4mm) (arrow-head). Signal intensity of the myocardium is identical to the skeletal muscle. Cine gradient-echo image (TE = 12) in the four chamber view (**B**) confirms the massive atrial enlargement as well as uniformly hindered diastolic ventricular filling. Flow void in systole within the left atrium is consistent with severe mitral valve regurgitation (arrow). Endomyocardial biopsy performed in the right ventricle revealed moderate interstitial fibrosis, immature elastic fibers and focal myocite hypertrophy and atrophy consistent with idiopathic restrictive cardiomyopathy.

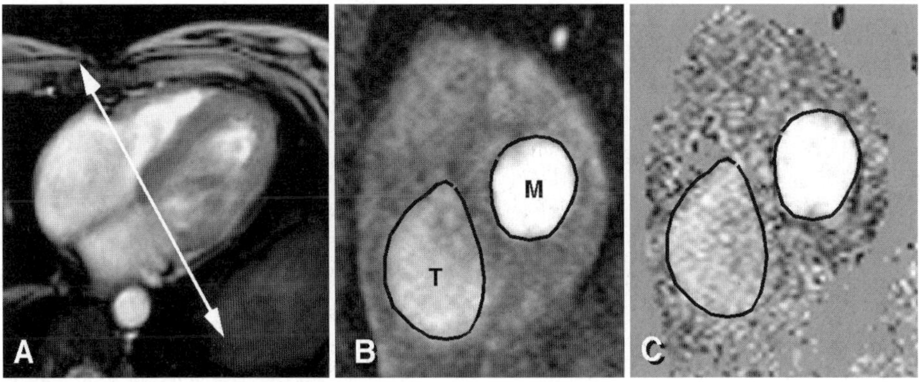

Fig. 6.**16** Restrictive cardiomyopathy.
Cine gradient-echo image in the four chamber view (**A**) shows the plane realized to analyze the flow within the atrioventricular valves (double arrow) perpendicular to the atrioventricular annuli. Velocity-encoded cine MR sequences reconstructed in magnitude (**B**), and in phase (**C**) allow the measurement of tricuspid (T) and mitral (M) flows.

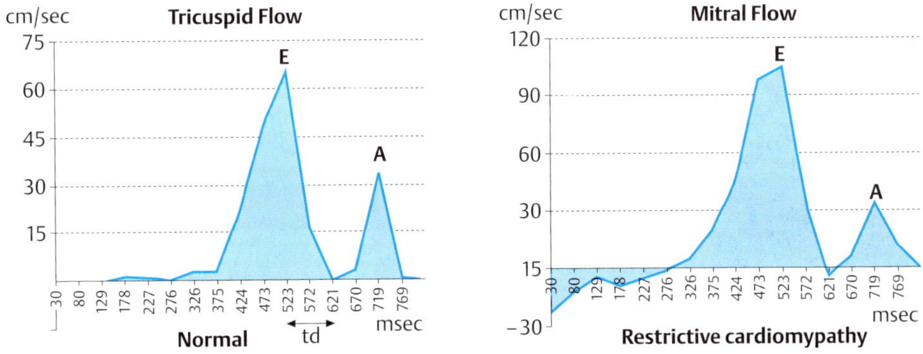

Fig. 6.**17** Restrictive cardiomyopathy.
Graphs of normal tricuspid flow (left) and mitral flow in a patient with restrictive cardiomyopathy (right) obtained on phase images performed perpendicular to the tricuspid and mitral annuli. The ventricular filling curves obtained are similar to the Doppler curves and show the same modifications of the E and A waves in case of restrictive cardiomyopathy. Presence of mitral regurgitation, increased early diastolic filling velocity (E wave ≥ 1.0 m/s), decreased atrial filling velocity (A wave ≤ 0.5 m/s), increased E/A ratio (≥ 2.0), decreased E wave deceleration time (td) (≤ 50 ms).

6.2.2 Endomyocardial Fibrosis

Endomyocardial fibrosis is a restrictive form of cardiomyopathy that results in impaired ventricular filling in diastole due to a non-compliant ventricle whereas systolic function remains normal, at least early in the disease. It may affect either one or both ventricles and it is particularly frequent in equatorial Africa. Its cause remains unknown and it is often associated with eosinophilia. It is characterized by fibrous endocardial thickening involving the inflow portion of the ventricles, the papillary muscles, chordae tendinae and the atrioventricular valves responsible for valvular regurgitation. Fibrosis may obliterate the apex of the ventricles with a mass of fibrous tissue, thrombus and calcifications. Surgery, consisting of resection of the fibrotic endocardium and replacing the mitral and/or tricuspid valves improves the survival [17]. As all restrictive cardiomyopathies, the major clinical challenge is to distinguish endomyocardial fibrosis from constrictive pericarditis because the clinical presentations may be similar. Regurgitant murmur is common in endomyocardial fibrosis whereas it is uncommon in constrictive pericarditis. 2D and Doppler echocardiography provide criteria for distinguishing the two conditions. Presence of mitral or tricuspid regurgitation, narrowing of the right and/or left cavities by echogenic material involving the apex or the inflow tract and papillary muscle with trabecular aspect favor endomyocardial fibrosis. But echocardiography does not provide accurate assessment of pericardial thickness and is limited in grading the extent of endomyocardial fibrosis, particularly in the right ventricle [18]. MRI is very effective to demonstrate the absence of pericardial thickening on spin-echo images (pericardial thick-

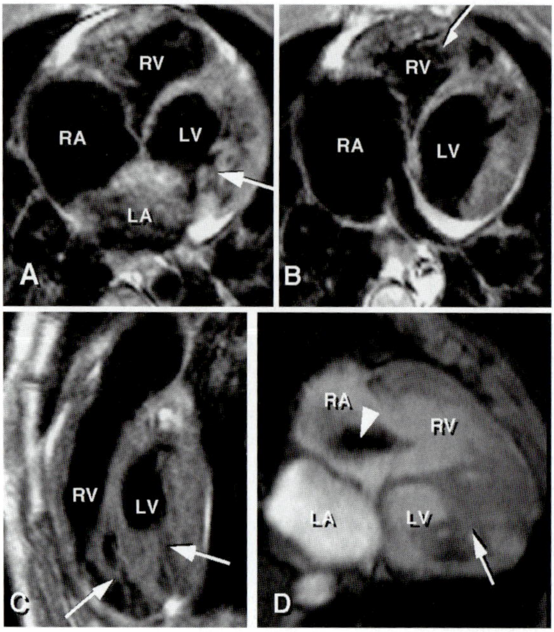

Fig. 6.**18** Endomyocardial fibrosis. T1 weighted spin-echo transverse (**A**, **B**) and sagittal (**C**) images show dilated right atrium (RA) and thickened trabeculated endocardial tissue involving the right (RV) and left (LV) ventricles (arrows). There is apical obliteration of both ventricles, particularly severe in the apex of LV and extending along the lateral wall and the septum. A substantial signal in the left atrial (LA) cavity is consistent with stasis of blood. Cine gradient-echo image (**D**) in the four chamber plane demonstrated exclusion of the LV apex (arrow), restricted diastolic ventricular filling and abnormal motion of the ventricular septum. Flow void in systole in the right atrium (arrow-head) is consistent with severe tricuspid valve regurgitation and pulmonary hypertension.

ness ≤ 4 mm). CT is particularly effective to detect the presence of linear calcifications along the inner border of the myocardium [19]. MRI, with its multiplanar capability allows direct visualization and mapping of endomyocardial fibrosis. The ventricular cavities, particularly the apex are often obliterated by extensive endocardial trabeculated tissue that may show a different signal as compared to adjacent normal myocardium [20]. Cine gradient-echo images provide additional information such as tricuspid or mitral flow void corresponding to atrioventricular valve regurgitation and abnormal ventricular diastolic filling pattern (Fig. 6.**18**). Endomyocardial biopsy may reveal fibrous tissue involving the endocardium and extending into the myocardium.

6.2.3 Spongy Myocardium

The persistence of spongy myocardium, also known as non-compaction of the ventricular myocardium, is a rare form of cardiomyopathy. During embryonic development, the heart consists of a trabecular network of sponge-like myocardium. Normally, as the heart develops, the myocardium becomes compacted and the mesh-like pattern disappears. This congenital disorder is characterized by the arrest of compaction of the loose myocardial meshwork during fetal development resulting in persistence of trabecular myocardium. The gross anatomic appearance is characterized by numerous, excessively prominent trabeculations and deep intertrabecular recesses. It may involve both the right and left ventricles but the reported cases are more frequent in the left ventricle. Other associated cardiac anomalies are frequently reported,

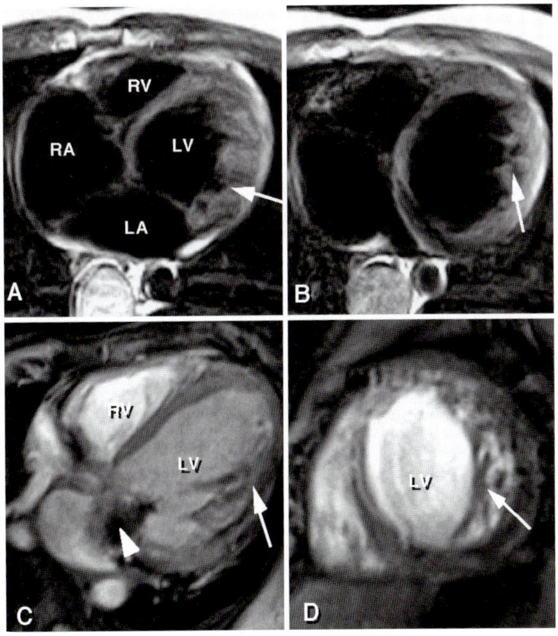

Fig. 6.**19** Spongy myocardium. T1-weighted transverse spin-echo images (**A**, **B**) show prominent trabeculations in the apex of the left ventricle (LV) (arrows) extending along the lateral wall. A substantial signal between the trabeculations is consistent with stasis of blood. Cine gradient-echo images in the four chamber (**C**) and short axis (**D**) planes demonstrated apical hypokinesia (ejection fraction: 45%), mitral regurgitation (arrow-head), numerous trabeculations in the apex and blood-filled recess in the lateral wall of the left ventricle (arrows).

including pulmonary atresia and coronary artery abnormalities. Isolated non-compaction of the left ventricle is extremely rare [21]. Clinical presentation includes signs of heart failure, arrhythmias and systemic embolization due to possible development of mural thrombi in the trabecular recesses. The decreased ventricular systolic function may be related to faulty intramural perfusion due to the presence of trabeculations and the decreased diastolic function may be due to abnormal ventricular compliance. 2D echocardiography reveals prominent trabeculations and deep intertrabecular recesses in the ventricular wall, particularly at the apex. MRI confirms these numerous trabeculations and deep recesses, sometimes blood- or clot-filled, in the apicolateral and apicoinferior regions of the left ventricle. Stasis of blood between trabeculations and in recesses may result in the presence of an intracavitary signal, reinforcing on T2-weighted images [22]. Cine gradient-echo images demonstrate flow in the deep recesses and allow evaluation of regional and global cardiac function (Fig. 6.**19**).

6.2.4 Hypertrophic Cardiomyopathy – Asymmetric

Hypertrophic cardiomyopathy (HC) is characterized by the presence of hypertrophied and non-dilated left ventricles without history of disease that could be responsible for ventricular hypertrophy. It may affect the right ventricle as well. Hypertrophic cardiomyopathy is classified as symmetric or asymmetric according to the location and extent of the hypertrophy. Asymmetric septal hypertrophy is the most frequent subtype of hypertrophic cardiomyopathy. It is characterized by a thickened ventricular

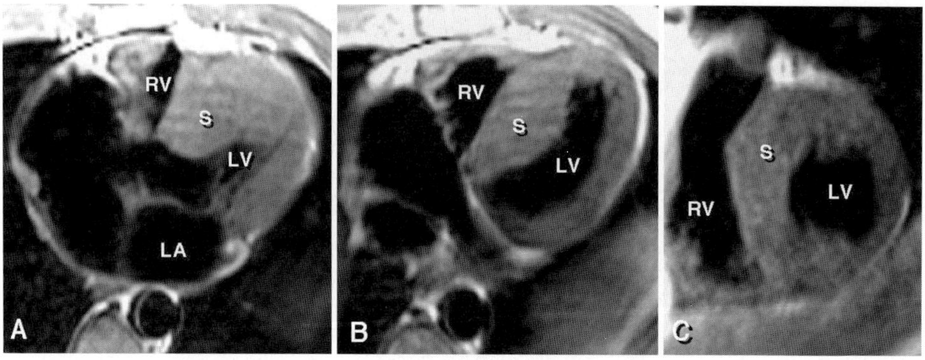

Fig. 6.**20** Asymmetric hypertrophic cardiomyopathy.
T1-weighted Spin-echo images show massive hypertrophy of the ventricular septum (S) (thickness: 26 mm) whereas the lateral wall of the left ventricle is normal (thickness: 12 mm). The entire septal wall is involved.

septum (≥ 15 mm) whereas the posterolateral wall of the left ventricle is not affected. It may be responsible for an obstruction of the left ventricular outflow tract as demonstrated by Doppler echocardiography and catheterization by a systolic subaortic pressure gradient. Doppler echocardiography is the procedure of choice to evaluate asymmetric hypertrophic cardiomyopathy. MRI has advantages over echocardiography including a larger field of view and better delineation of the pathology. It better demonstrates the distribution, extent and severity of the hypertrophic process [23]. On spin-echo images, the exact measurement of the septal wall thickness compared to the posterolateral wall as well as myocardial mass can be carried out (Fig. 6.**20**). Cine MRI provides excellent evaluation of cardiac function. It can also document the anterior displacement of the mitral valve during systole (systolic anterior motion; SAM) as well as the left ventricular outflow tract obstruction characterized by the presence of a flow void in the subaortic region during systole and the severity of frequently associated mitral regurgitation (Fig. 6.**21**). But there is no correlation between the distribution and severity of the hypertrophic process and the degree of obstruction as compared with catheterization data. On the other hand, the importance of the subaortic flow void due to turbulence and high velocities and its distribution during systole is a qualitative index of the degree of obstruction. Velocity-encoded cine MRI can provide measurement of the exact degree of obstruction, like Doppler echocardiography, by calculation of the maximum velocity within the outflow tract and by using modified Bernoulli equation.

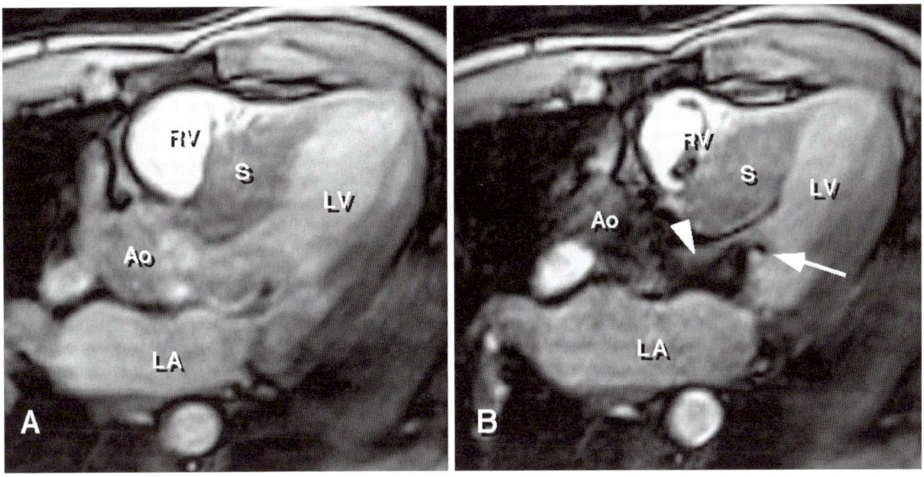

Fig. 6.**21** Asymmetric hypertrophic cardiomyopathy (same patient as Fig. 6.**20**).
Cine gradient-echo images in the long axis plane confirm septal hypertrophy (S) on diastolic (**A**) as well as on systolic (**B**) images. Cardiac function was normal (ejection fraction = 69%). A flow void emanating from the subaortic region during systole (arrow-head on **B**) and systolic anterior motion of the mitral valve (arrow) without mitral regurgitation are also demonstrated. Velocity-encoded cine images centered on the left ventricular outflow tract allowed the measurement of a V_{max} of 2.5 m/s corresponding to a subaortic gradient of 25 mm Hg.

6.2.5 Hypertrophic Cardiomyopathy – Symmetric

Symmetric hypertrophic cardiomyopathy is a primary myocardial disease characterized by the presence of hypertrophied and non-dilated left ventricles without history of disease that could be responsible for this ventricular hypertrophy. It is frequently familial, transmitted genetically. It may affect the right ventricle as well. In symmetric hypertrophic cardiomyopathy (concentric), the hypertrophic process involves all parts of the myocardial wall in the same proportion and is responsible for small diastolic cavity dimensions, a decreased ventricular compliance in diastole and a hyperdynamic systolic function leading to cavity obliteration. Doppler echocardiography is the procedure of choice to evaluate symmetric hypertrophic cardiomyopathy [24]. MRI has advantages over echocardiography including a larger field of view and better delineation of the pathology. With its multiplanar capability, it better demonstrates the distribution, extent and severity of the hypertrophic process [25]. On spin-echo images, the exact measurement of the wall thickness as well as myocardial mass can be performed. Cine MRI provides excellent evaluation of systolic and diastolic cardiac function and the severity of potentially associated mitral regurgitation. A subaortic flow void due to turbulence and high velocities may be encountered without a significant gradient due to the rapid emptying of the left ventricle during systole (Fig. 6.**22**).

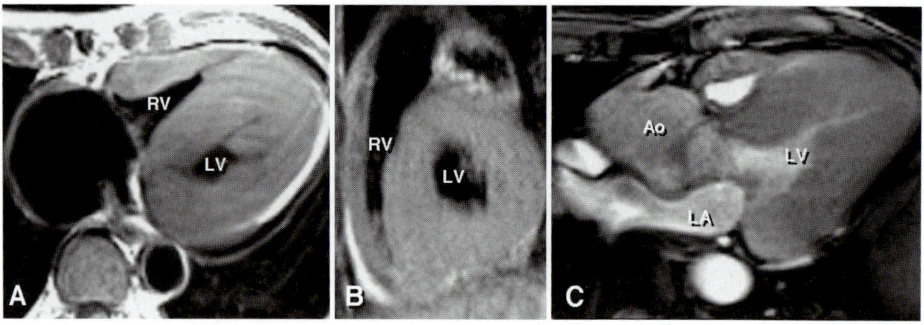

Fig. 6.**22** Symmetric hypertrophic cardiomyopathy.
T1-weighted transverse (**A**) and sagittal (**B**) spin-echo images show marked symmetric hypertrophy of the entire left ventricle wall (thickness: 25 mm). The cavity is almost obliterated. Cine gradient-echo images in the long axis plane (**C**) demonstrate hyperdynamic cardiac systolic function (EF = 75%) and complete obliteration of the left ventricular cavity (LV) in systole.

6.2.6 Biventricular Hypertrophic Cardiomyopathy

Hypertrophic cardiomyopathy may affect the right ventricle as well. In biventricular hypertrophic cardiomyopathy, the hypertrophic process involves all parts of the myocardial wall in the same proportion and is responsible for small diastolic cavity dimensions, decreased right and left ventricular compliances in diastole and a hyperdynamic systolic function leading to cavity obliteration. When the right ventricle is involved, a right ventricular outflow tract obstruction may exist, potentially severe. Doppler echocardiography is the procedure of choice to evaluate biventricular hypertrophic cardiomyopathy. MRI has advantages over echocardiography including a larger field of view and better delineation of the pathology. With its multiplanar capability, it better demonstrates the distribution, extent and severity of the hypertrophic process. On spin-echo images, the exact measurement of the wall thickness as well as myocardial mass can be performed. Cine MRI provides excellent evaluation of systolic and diastolic cardiac function and the severity of potentially associated atrioventricular valve regurgitation (Fig. 6.**23**). A flow void in the right ventricular outflow tract due to turbulence and high velocities may be encountered with a significant gradient due to the obstruction created by right ventricular hypertrophy. Velocity-encoded cine MRI can provide measurement of the exact degree of obstruction, like Doppler echocardiography, by calculation of the maximum velocity within the right outflow tract and by using modified Bernoulli equation.

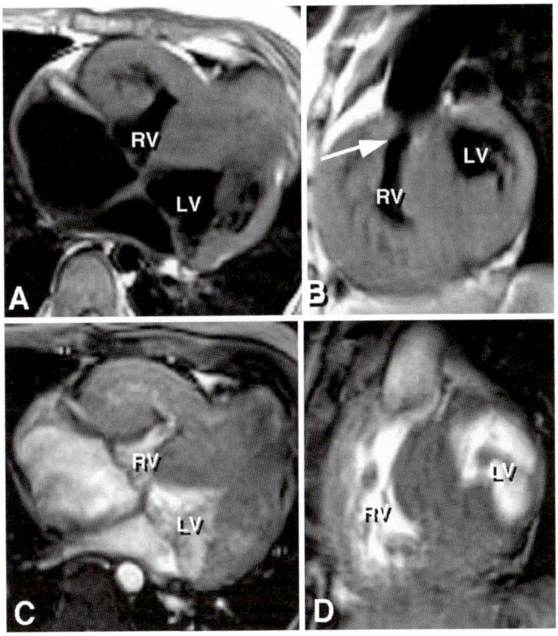

Fig. 6.**23** Biventricular hypertrophic cardiomyopathy. T1-weighted transverse (**A**) and sagittal (**B**) spin-echo images show marked hypertrophy of both the right (RV) and left (LV) ventricles. The left cavity is almost obliterated. A marked hypertrophy of the right ventricular outflow tract is responsible for severe subpulmonary stenosis. (arrow on **B**). Cine gradient-echo images in the four chamber (**C**) and sagittal (**D**) planes demonstrated severe impaired diastolic filling and a tight stenosis of the right ventricular outflow tract. It was confirmed on the sagittal velocity-encoded cine sequence with a maximum velocity of 5 m/s, corresponding to a subpulmonary gradient of 100 mm Hg.

6.2.7 Apical Hypertrophic Cardiomyopathy and Double-Chambered Left Ventricle

Hypertrophic cardiomyopathy can be localized at the apex and in this case is defined by a disproportionate hypertrophy of the apical region of the left ventricle with normal thickness of the basal segments. MRI is of major value for assessing the degree of myocardial hypertrophy exclusively localized at the apex, particularly with the long axis and the four chamber views [26] (Fig. 6.**24**).

A double-chambered left ventricle is a rare anomaly of unknown etiology characterized by the subdivision of the left ventricular cavity by an anomalous septum or muscle bundle (Fig. 6.**25**). It is associated with endocardial fibroelastosis and presumed cardiomyopathy. It could represent the end stage of a hypertrophic cardiomyopathy localized to the midportion of the left ventricle [27]. It has to be differentiated from congenital aneurysms and diverticulae. The left ventricle is poorly contractile and mitral regurgitation is common. The prognosis of this anomaly is very poor.

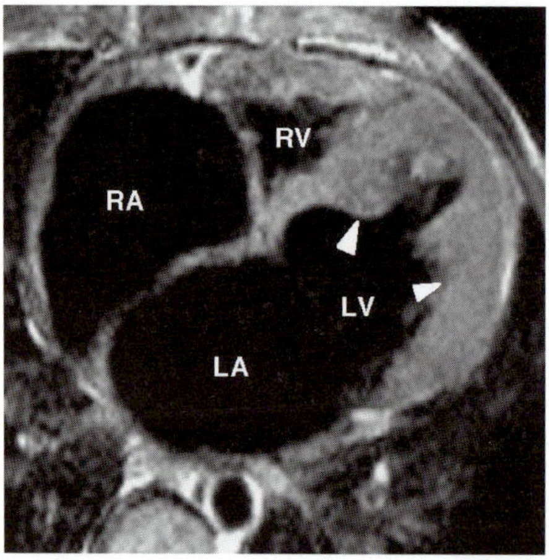

Fig. 6.**24**: Apical hypertrophic cardiomyopathy.
T1-weighted transverse spin-echo image shows hypertrophy of the apical region of the left ventricle (arrow-heads) with normal thickness of the basal segments.

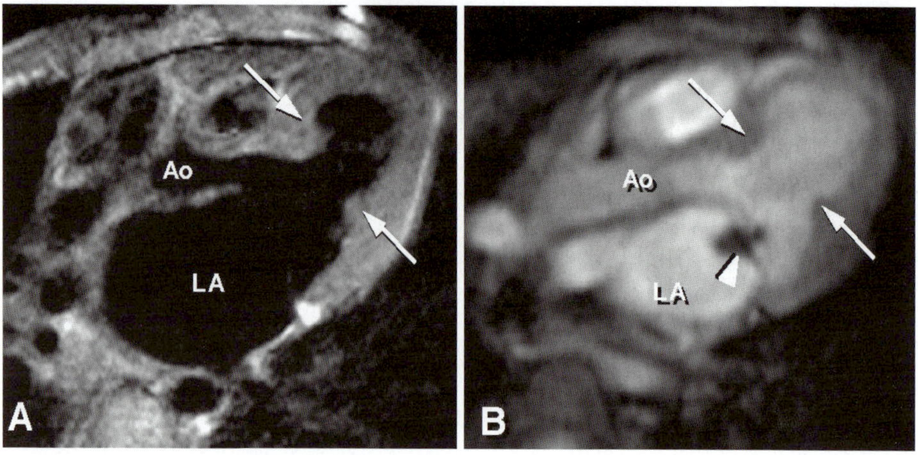

Fig. 6.**25** Double-chambered left ventricle.
Transverse spin-echo (**A**) and cine gradient-echo (**B**) images demonstrate the subdivision of the left ventricular cavity by an anomalous septum or muscle bundle (arrows) and a flow void within the left atrium (LA) corresponding to mitral regurgitation (arrow-head).

6.2.8 Dilated Cardiomyopathy

Dilated cardiomyopathy is the most common cause of cardiomyopathies. It is characterized by the enlargement of one or both ventricles and systolic dysfunction (usually affecting the left ventricle) and exclusion of other conditions that cause ventricular dilatation. In 20 to 30% of cases, familial inheritance can be demonstrated, with autosomal dominant as the most common mode of transmission. Dilated cardiomyopathy can exist either as a primary disorder or as a complication of or in association with other conditions: myopathies and systemic disorders including metabolic

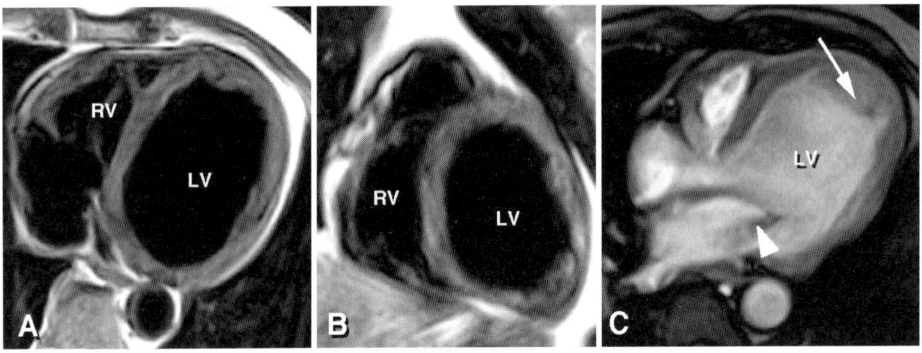

Fig. 6.**26** Dilated cardiomyopathy.
T1-weighted spin-echo images (**A**, **B**) show marked uniform dilatation of the left ventricular cavity (LV). Cine gradient-echo images in the four chamber view (**C**) demonstrate severe global impaired systolic function with an ejection fraction of 35% and a flow void emanating from the left atrioventricular valve during systole consistent with a mild mitral regurgitation (arrow-head). Low to medium signal intensity mass at the apex of the left ventricle is consistent of thrombus (arrow).

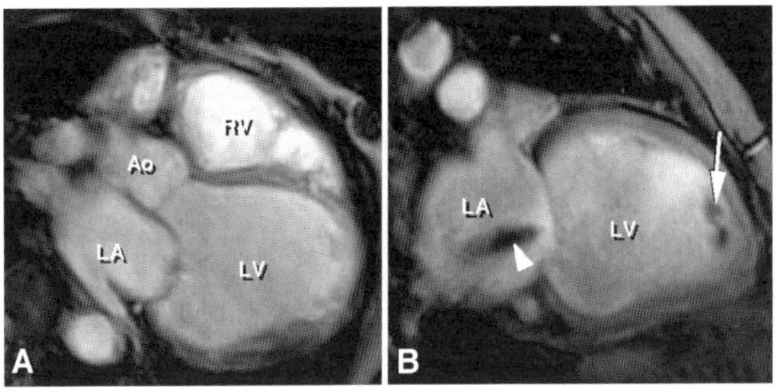

Fig. 6.**27** Dilated cardiomyopathy. Cine gradient-echo images in the long axis (**A**) and two chamber (**B**) views show massive and uniform dilatation of the left ventricular cavity (LV) and mitral regurgitation (arrow-head). Thrombus at the apex of the left ventricle is obvious. Usually but not always, thrombus appears as a low signal intensity mass on cine gradient-echo images.

deficiencies, immunologic abnormalities or myocarditis [28]. Echocardiography is the procedure of choice to evaluate dilated cardiomyopathy. MRI has advantages over echocardiography including a larger field of view and better depiction of the morphology and contractility of the affected ventricle and can be used to monitor the progression of the disease and the response to therapy as well as for the detection of the often associated thrombi. On spin-echo images, the exact measurement of the wall thickness as well as myocardial mass can be carried out. The left ventricle is often markedly dilated and its geometry is altered. The right ventricle can be dilated as well. The thickness of the left ventricular wall is usually normal but there is a substantial increase in left ventricular mass. Cine MRI provides excellent evaluation of global and regional systolic and diastolic cardiac function and demonstrates usually global hypokinesia with a severe decrease of the ejection fraction. Functional mitral and/or tricuspid regurgitation is often encountered due to annulus dilatation. Cine MRI can be used to assess its severity [29] (Fig. 6.**26**). MRI can detect associated thrombi in atria and ventricles, particularly on cine images, which are some times difficult to visualize with echocardiography (Fig. 6.**27**).

6.3 References

1. Stark DD, Higgins CB, Lanzer P, et al. Magnetic resonance imaging of the pericardium: Normal and pathologic findings. Radiology 1984; 150: 469–474.
2. Sechtem U, Tscholakoff D, Higgins CB. MRI of the normal pericardium. AJR 1986; 147: 239–244.
3. McMurdo KK, Webb WR, von Schulthess GK, Gamsu G. Magnetic resonance imaging of the superior pericardial recesses. AJR 1985; 145: 985–988.
4. Sechtem U, Tscholakoff D, Higgins CB. MRI of the abnormal pericardium. AJR 1986; 147: 245–252.
5. Frank H, Globits S. Magnetic resonance imaging evaluation of myocardial and pericardial disease. J. Magn Reson Imaging 1999; 10: 617–626.
6. Mehta A, Mehta M, Jain AC. Constrictive pericarditis. Clin Cardiol 1999; 22: 334–344.
7. Fowler NO. Constrictive pericarditis; its history and current status. Clin Cardiol 1995; 18: 341–350.
8. Oh JK, Hatle LK, Seward JB, et al. Diagnostic role of Doppler echocardiography in constrictive pericarditis. J Am Coll Cardiol 1994; 23: 154–162.
9. Soulen RL, Stark DD, Higgins CB. Magnetic resonance imaging of constrictive pericardial disease. Am J Cardiol 1985; 55: 480–484.
10. Masui T, Finck S, Higgins CB. Constrictive pericarditis and restrictive cardiomyopathy: evaluation with MR imaging. Radiology 1992; 182: 369–373.
11. Barakos J, Brown J, Higgins CB. Magnetic resonance imaging of secondary cardiac and paracardiac masses. AJR 1989; 153: 47–50.
12. Kushwaha SS, Fallon JT, Fluster V. Restrictive cardiomyopathy. N Engl J Med 1997; 336: 267–276.
13. Zieman SJ, Fortuin NJ. Hypertrophic and restrictive cardiomyopathies in the elderly. Cardiology Clinics 1999; 17: 159–172.
14. Sechtem U, Higgins CB, Sommerhoff BA, et al. Magnetic resonance imaging of restrictive cardiomyopathy. Am J Cardiol 1987; 59: 480–482.
15. Appleton CP, Hatle LK, Popp RL. Demonstration of restrictive ventricular physiology by Doppler echocardiography. J Am Coll Cardiol 1988; 11: 757–768.
16. Celletti F, Fattori R, Napoli G, et al. Assessment of restrictive cardiomyopathy of amyloid or idiopathic etiology by magnetic resonance imaging. Am J Cardiol 1999; 83: 798–801.
17. Gupta P, Valiathan M, Balakrishnan K, et al. Clinical course of endomyocardial fibrosis. Br Heart J 1989; 62:450–454.
18. Acquatella H, Schiller N, Puigbo J, et al. Value of two-dimensional echocardiography in endomyocardial disease with and without eosinophilia: a clinical and pathologic study. Circulation 1983; 67: 1219–1226.
19. Mousseaux E, Hernigou A, Azencot M, et al. Endomyocardial fibrosis; electron-beam CT features. Radiology 1996; 198: 755–760.

20. D'Silva SA, Kholi A, Dalvi BV, et al. MRI in right ventricular endomyocardial fibrosis. Am Heart J 1992; 123: 1390–1392.
21. Ichida F, Hamamichi Y, Miyawaki T, et al. Clinical features of isolated noncompaction of the ventricular myocardium. J Am Coll Cardiol 1999; 34: 233–240.
22. Hany TF, Jenni R, Debatin JF. MR appearance of isolated noncompaction of the left ventricle. JMRI 1997; 7: 437–438.
23. Arrive L, Assayag P, Russ G, et al. MRI and cine MRI of asymmetric septal hypertrophic cardiomyopathy. J Comput Assist Tomogr 1994; 718: 376–382.
24. Pons-Llado G, Carreras F, Borras X, et al. Comparison of morphologic assessment of hypertrophic cardiomyopathy by magnetic resonance versus echocardiographic imaging. Am J Cardiol 1997; 79: 1651–1656.
25. Park JH, Kim YM, Chung JW, et al. MR imaging of hypertrophic cardiomyopathy. Radiology 1992; 185: 441–446.
26. Soler R, Rodriguez E, Rodriguez JA, et al. Magnetic resonance imaging of apical hypertrophic cardiomyopathy. J Thorac Imaging 1997; 12: 221–225.
27. Caron KH, Hernandez RJ, Goble M, Beekman R. MR imaging of double chambered left ventricle. J Comput Assist Tomogr 1991; 15: 140–142.
28. Bachinski LL, Roberts R. Causes of dilated cardiomyopathy. Cardiology Clinics 1998; 16: 603–610.
29. Fujita N, Hartiala J, O'Sullivan M, et al. Assessment of left ventricular diastolic function in dilated cardiomyopathy with cine MRI: effect of an angiotensin converting enzyme inhibitor, benazepril. Am Heart J 1993; 125: 171–177.

7 Ischemic Heart Disease

This chapter reviews MR imaging techniques used to evaluate ischemic heart disease and discusses the advantages and limitations of these techniques for providing clinically useful information in the assessment of coronary artery disease (CAD).

7.1 Imaging and Analysis Techniques

The different imaging modalities used for the evaluation of coronary artery disease include dynamic cine imaging techniques providing functional information on regional and global myocardial dysfunction, myocardial perfusion imaging techniques that provide relative differences in regional myocardial blood flow distribution and, when used in combination with a stress test, the latter provides estimates of coronary flow reserve. Recent progress in fast imaging techniques and high resolution MRA provide adequate image quality for visualization of the coronary artery. The accuracy and reproducibility of these MRA techniques for routine investigation of coronary lesions is still limited, but new high-field-strength clinical magnets, high-performance gradient hardware, and ultrafast pulse sequence technology are rapidly making the vision of a comprehensive "one-stop shop" cardiac MR imaging examination of CAD a reality [1].

7.1.1 Dynamic Cine Imaging Techniques

Gated cine images obtained in different planes across the cardiac chambers allow the evaluation of global and regional wall motions and contraction anomalies [2]. Dynamic imaging techniques and standardized anatomic imaging planes are described in Chapter 1. Several breath-hold sequences can be applied to adequately visualize ventricular wall motion. MR images provide the unique characteristic of high tissue differentiation and high blood to myocardium contrast allowing not only a perfect assessment of wall motion and ventricular cavity but also accurate evaluation of myocardial wall thickening.

7.1.2 Quantitative Analysis of LV Function

Using multi-slice cine MR imaging techniques, the three-dimensional geometry of the heart can be imaged at high temporal and spatial resolution [3]. As a tomographic imaging technique, volumetric measurements do not rely on any geometric assumptions and therefore are more accurate for both normal and abnormal ventricular

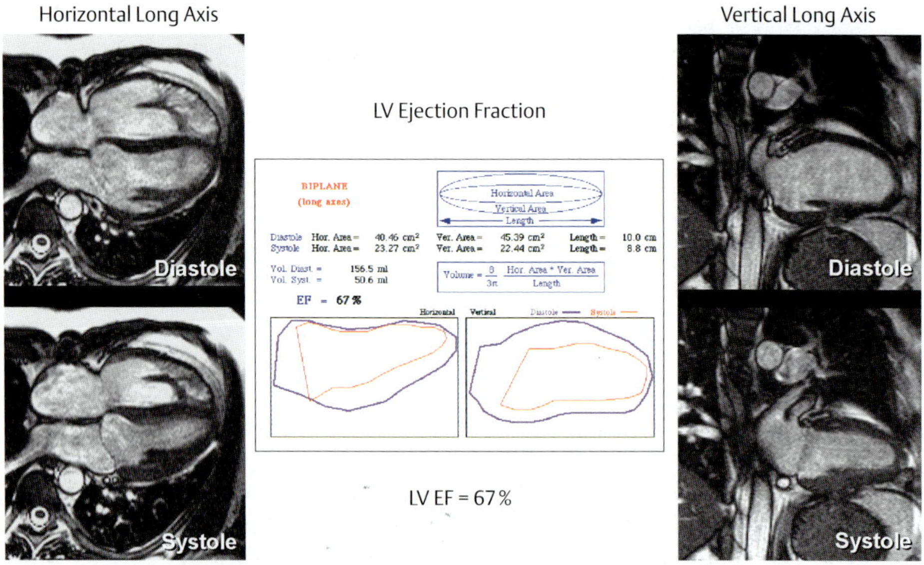

Fig. 7.**1** Left ventricular ejection fraction calculated from two orthogonal cine sequences along the cardiac long axis; Horizontal long axis (left) and vertical long axis (right). The ejection fraction is calculated using the biplane area-length geometric approximation.

anatomy. Oblique MRI acquisitions, in particular in the short-axis orientation, have proved their usefulness for the determination of left ventricular wall motion alterations. High contrast MR images allow the assessment of not only wall motion, but also wall thickening and differentiation of systolic and diastolic functions. It has been shown that wall-thickening analysis is more sensitive in the detection of dysfunctional myocardium than wall motion analysis.

The most commonly used parameter used for the evaluation of left ventricular function is the global ejection fraction (EF) calculated from the ratio of LV volumes in diastole and systole. In the normal left ventricle, geometric assumptions based on the elliptical shape of the ventricle have been validated in projectional images from X-ray angiography and tomographic planes along the cardiac main axes in echocardiography. These single-plane or biplane geometric formulae can also be used in cine MR images for accurate and reproducible assessment of left ventricular ejection fraction. Typical geometric formulae using the area-length technique (see Fig. 7.**1**) can be applied in ventricles that have reasonably elliptical shapes. However, in ventricles that have distorted geometric shapes secondary to severe myocardial infarctions or ischemia-induced regional wall motion anomalies, the geometric assumptions are prone to significant errors. In these cases, a more accurate measurement of ventricular volumes will require more detailed imaging of the heart through contiguous three-dimensional volume acquisitions. Dynamic cine MR imaging in multiple planes, in particular in contiguous short axis planes from the base of the heart to the apex (see

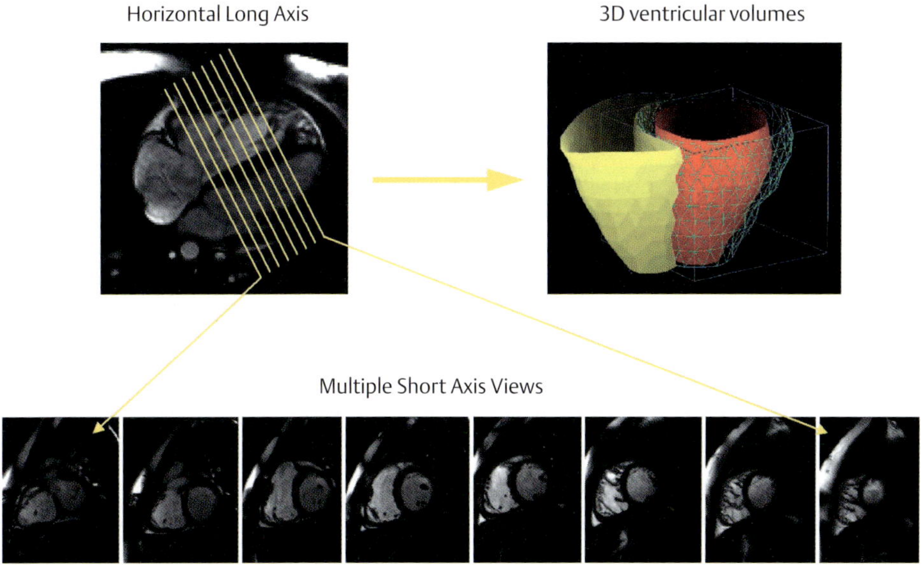

Fig. 7.2 Assessment of ventricular function and volumes from series of contiguous short axis cine images.

Fig. 7.2) have proven to be more accurate in the determination of ventricular regional wall parameters.

7.1.3 Myocardial Tagging Techniques

Myocardial tagging is an MR imaging method that uses a sequence of RF pulses to presaturate thin planes of myocardium prior to imaging. These "tags" persist in the myocardium through the heart cycle and can be used to track motion of the heart by acquiring images perpendicular to the tagging planes (Fig. 7.3). Quantitative measurements of strain pattern changes require determination of precise tag position by using tag detection algorithms. Post-processing software can be used to obtain highly accurate estimates of tag displacement [4]. Three-dimensional strain patterns provide detailed strain maps of the entire left ventricle in both time and space. MRI tagging of the myocardium is a powerful method for the assessment of mechanical function of the myocardium and contributes significantly in the understanding of the normal and abnormal physiology of myocardial contractility and fiber shortening. It is a very powerful method for the assessment of mechanical alterations in settings of ischemia, infarction, myocardial stunning post-ischemia, myocardial hibernation after chronic or recurrent ischemia, and in the setting of post-infarction left ventricular remodeling. Quantitative analysis of tagged images is usually relatively complex, requiring significant manual interactions and generates a very large amount of data. Thus, the development of effective software analysis packages incorporating automated or semi-

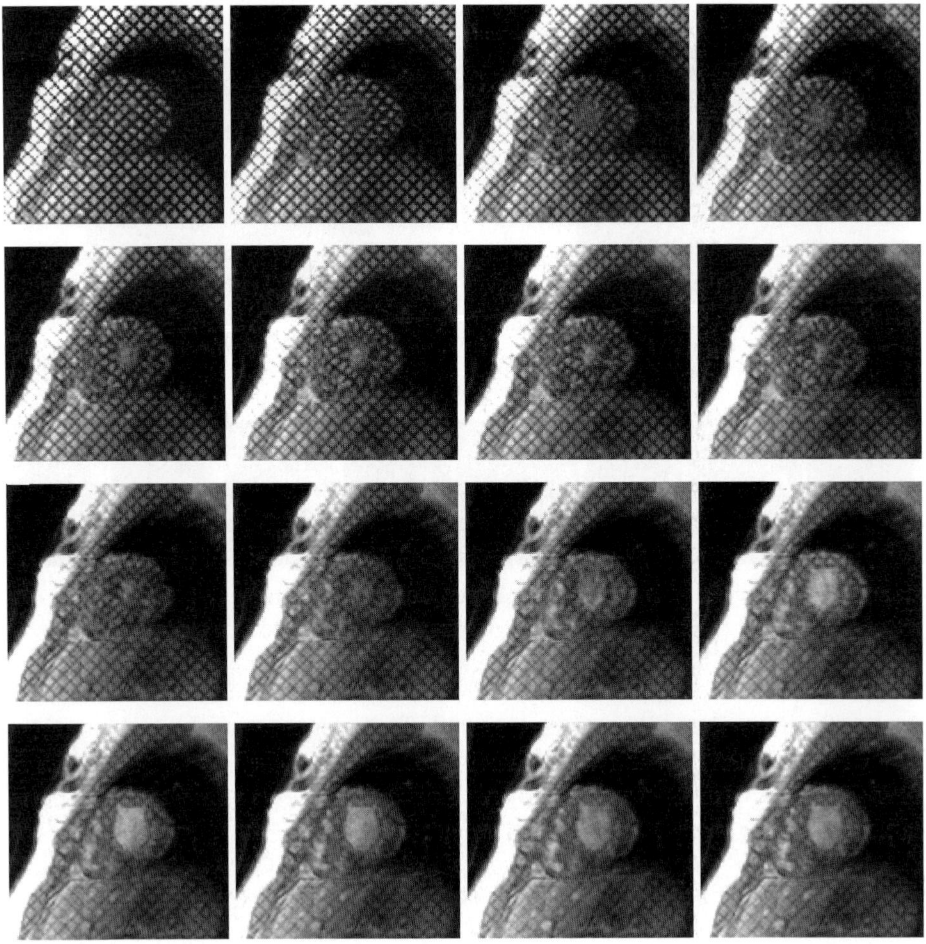

Fig. 7.**3** Example of "tagged" short axis cine images. Notice how the presaturated cross-lines fade out over time from the beginning to the end of the heart cycle.

automated image analysis techniques represents an important aspect of the recent development in this technique by academic and commercial development groups. Despite substantial development in this area, further development is badly needed in reducing the effort of skilled observers in image analysis and data manipulation, as well as for facilitating more rapid and flexible data display and interpretation if this approach is to be widely adopted in clinical applications.

7.1.4 Myocardial Perfusion Imaging Techniques

First-pass myocardial perfusion imaging techniques are rapidly emerging as a powerful tool for evaluation of rest and stress changes in myocardial blood flow alterations. Contrast-enhanced first-pass perfusion imaging uses T1-weighted pulse sequences that result in myocardial brightening compared with the pre-gadolinium images [5]. The simple explanation of the dynamics of myocardial gadolinium uptake based on a single-compartment model at equilibrium is based on the assumption that contrast enhancement is dependent on myocardial perfusion and not on contrast entry into the myocytes (Fig. 7.**4**). In general, normal myocardium will appear bright while infarcted myocardium and areas of low coronary perfusion will appear dark with a lower signal intensity than normal myocardium on post-gadolinium images. If infarcted myocardium does not have a resting perfusion deficit, however, it may not exhibit a decreased signal [6].

Accurate and comprehensive evaluation of overall myocardial perfusion requires the acquisition of images over the entire heart with high temporal resolution to capture the first pass of contrast through the myocardium. This has been a serious limiting factor on early scanners that were only able to acquire a small number of imaging planes across the heart during the short transit time of the contrast agent. Advances in hardware and pulse sequence technology now allow the acquisition of

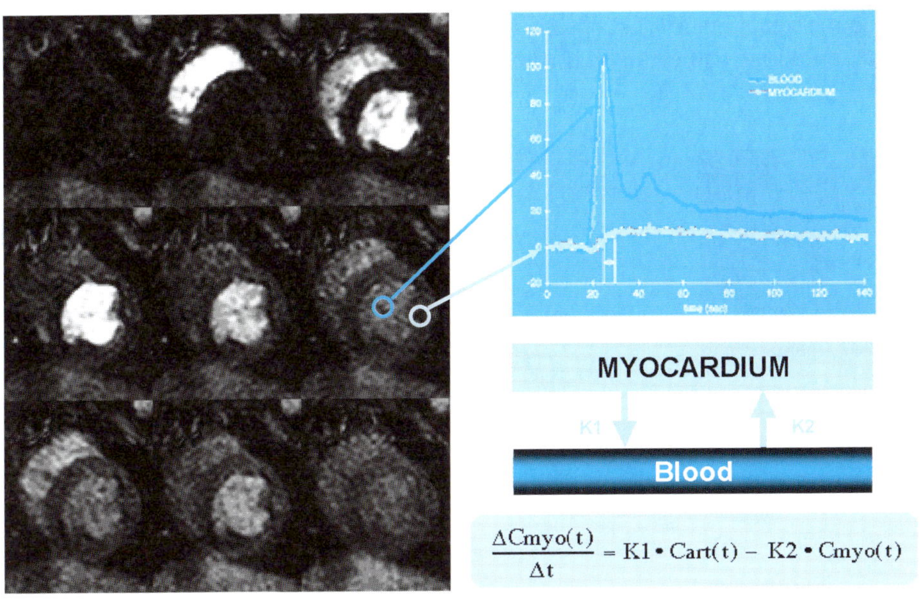

Fig. 7.**4** Sequence of images acquired during the first pass of contrast media across myocardial circulation. Intensity curves over the blood and myocardial area are used to estimate local myocardial perfusion using a simple diffusion compartmental model (by courtesy of J. P. Vallée, University Hospital of Geneva).

multiple imaging planes every heartbeat during the tracking of contrast agent bolus. An added advantage of single-heartbeat acquisition is that breath-holding may not be required during image acquisition. Trade-offs for higher image resolution can be made by reducing the temporal sampling rate. Segmentation to more than one heartbeat requires breath-holding, however.

7.1.5 Delayed Contrast Enhancement Imaging of Injured Myocardium

Numerous MR imaging sequences were shown to differentiate areas of myocardial injury with higher signal intensity than normal myocardium. Some early studies showed that T2-weighted MR sequences without contrast injection showed increased signal intensity in areas of myocardial infarction [7, 8]. More recent studies showed even higher specificity and sensitivity of gadolinium-enhanced MR imaging sequences showing late hyperenhancement of regions of irreversible myocardial injury post infarction (Fig. 7.5). Extensive comparisons of different imaging sequences [9] showed that the most promising technique that provides the highest spatial and contrast resolution between injured myocardium and normal myocardium is a breath-hold inversion-recovery segmented turbo fast low-angle (turbo-FLASH) T1-weighted sequence. Cardiac-specific imaging sequences based on these observations were recently introduced by most major manufacturers where the image acquisition is synchronized with diastole, and gradient-moment refocusing is used to reduce motion artifacts. In these sequences, the inversion time (TI) is specifically chosen to null the signal intensity of normal myocardium after contrast agent administration. After appropriate adjustment of the optimal TI delay for each individual patient

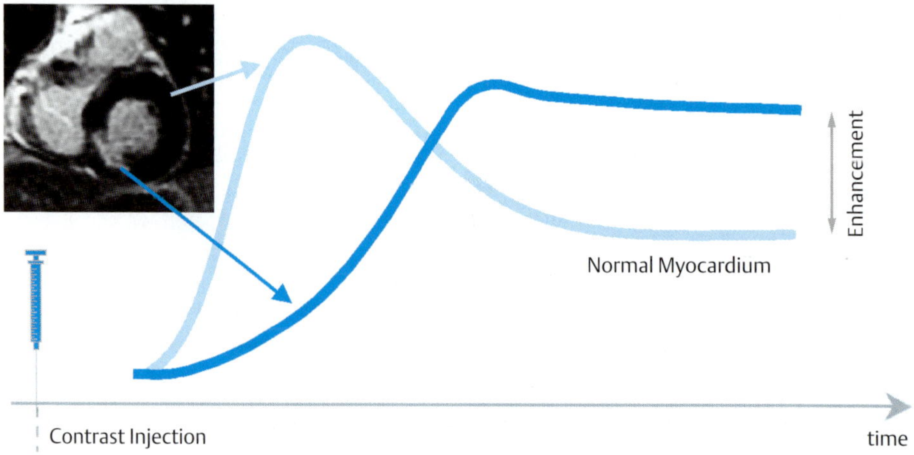

Fig. 7.5 The phenomenon of late enhancement results from different kinetics of contrast wash-in and wash-out curves in normal and irreversibly damaged myocardium where contrast persists for longer periods of time.

(usually between 200 and 300 msec), images are acquired 5–20 min after intravenous injection of 0.2 mmol/kg of gadolinium. For coverage of the entire heart, multiple single-section short axis images are acquired in 10 to 12 breath-hold acquisitions [10]. Faster acquisition techniques using higher performance gradients and three-dimensional acquisition techniques are also being developed to improve image acquisition and reduce the acquisition time.

7.1.6 High Resolution MR Angiography of Coronary Arteries

Coronary angiography with magnetic resonance imaging techniques is probably the most challenging and also most promising area of development in cardiac MRI today [11]. Various methods have been proposed to improve signal-to-noise and contrast-to-noise ratios while achieving the best possible spatial and temporal resolution. When time-of-flight MR angiography techniques were first introduced, two-dimensional (2D) breath-hold angiography was applied to the coronary arteries. Several variations of 2D gradient-echo techniques were proposed by different investigators for the visualization of coronary arteries. These techniques, while promising, relied on expert user placement of slices to cover the coronary arteries and suffered from poor through-plane resolution. With faster imaging techniques it became possible to acquire stacks of 2D coronary MRA with gradient-echo techniques obtained in the plane of each coronary vessel for improved resolution [12]. The 2D approach takes full advantage of the inflow-related contrast between coronary blood and surrounding stationary tissue. However, 2D approaches are often limited by the tortuous nature of the coronary vessels, the signal-to-noise ratio constraints and errors related to inconsistency between serial breath-holds. With the development of enhanced gradient systems and the improvement in image acquisition pulse sequences, respiratory-compensated 3D coronary MRA techniques became available (Fig. 7.**6**). 3D coronary MRA overcomes several of the limitations of 2D techniques and has significant advantages, including improved through-plane resolution and improved slice registration [13]. With 3D techniques, contiguous thin adjacent slices can be obtained and the image data can be post-processed in any oblique or curved orientation to better visualize the tortuous trajectory of coronary arteries. However, 3D coronary MRA often offers a lower contrast-to-noise ratio due to attenuated blood-inflow effects. Thus, the use of contrast agents for 3D coronary MRA techniques may have greater potential than in 2D approaches. Contrast agents shorten T1 and enhance blood signal, allowing the use of shorter TRs and decreasing the time required for image acquisition. Contrast-enhanced images are also less susceptible to signal loss due to slow flow, an artifact that could lead to overestimation of stenosis [14].

Among the major limitations of coronary MRA are the artifacts and misregistration errors resulting from respiratory motion. While the breath-hold technique may be successfully applicable in studies performed on healthy volunteers, it has serious limitations in clinical practice. Patients with cardiac or pulmonary disease frequently have difficulty sustaining adequate breath-holds, particularly for acquisitions exceed-

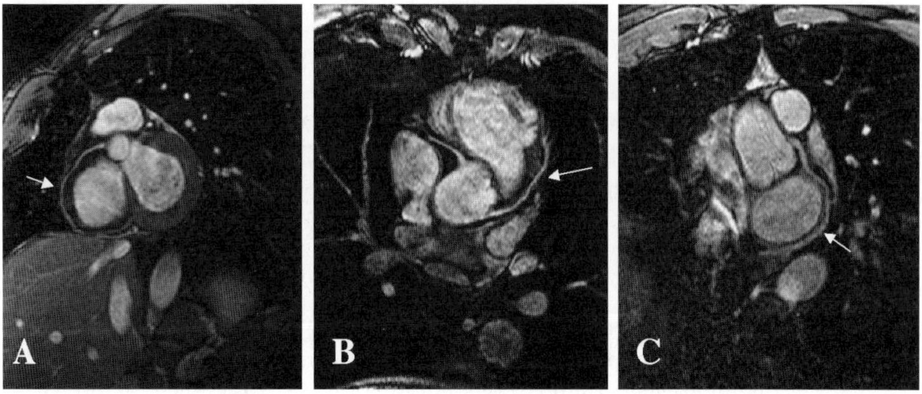

Fig. 7.**6** Images of coronary arteries obtained in different "thick-slab" oblique planes along the (**A**) right coronary artery, (**B**) the left anterior descending and (**C**) the circumflex arteries.

ing several seconds. The use of respiratory maneuvers such as hyperventilation and oxygen supplementation to facilitate and prolong breath-holding may not be applicable in all patients. Additionally, during prolonged breath-holds there is often a slight diaphragmatic drift that can induce changes in cardiac position of up to 1 cm resulting in significant registration errors. Misregistration results in apparent gaps between the segments of the visualized coronary arteries, which could be misinterpreted as signal voids from coronary stenosis. To overcome these limitations with breath-holding, several methods have been developed to allow for free-breathing coronary MRA. Respiratory belts have been used to monitor chest wall expansion and thereby gate image acquisition to the end-expiratory position. This technique is often not reliable due to inconsistency of respiratory gating and to the lack of a direct relationship between the chest wall expansion and the diaphragmatic motion. An alternative to respiratory gating was developed using MR navigators where the MR images are used to monitor diaphragmatic craniocaudal displacement. A vertical monitoring region of interest is positioned on the dome of the right diaphragm and diaphragmatic motion is used to gate coronary MRA acquisition. Images are typically acquired during expiration (minimal expansion) and the gating process can be either prospective (i.e., before data acquisition) or retrospective (i.e., following data acquisition, but before image reconstruction) [15]. Although navigator approaches greatly improve patient comfort and do not require significant subject collaboration, obtaining high-quality images requires the use of a narrow gating respiratory window and may significantly prolong the scan duration. This may be particularly impractical in contrast-enhanced coronary MRA sequences.

7.2 Assessment of Ventricular Function Alterations

7.2.1 Global and Regional Wall Motion Anomalies

Standard and breath-hold cine MR imaging provides accurate and highly reproducible measurements of left ventricular volumes, ejection fraction and myocardial mass. Since multiple tomographic images can be acquired encompassing the entire heart, measurement of volumes and mass are not dependent on the assumption of geometric models, as required with X-ray angiography and 2D-echocardiography (Fig. 7.**7**). In the presence of ventricular asymmetry caused by regional infarction and remodeling of the left ventricle, formulae for calculating volumes and masses from geometric models have questionable validity. With the ability to acquire imaging in multiple oblique planes, cine MR imaging techniques provide an ideal tool for accurate assessment of global and regional alteration in myocardial function in coronary artery disease. Changes in ventricular function and wall thickness post myocardial infarction can be accurately measured and visualized (Fig. 7.**8**). MRI provides a unique and highly accurate non-invasive technique to monitor changes in regional and global ventricular function following therapeutic interventions of coronary revascularization. It also allows the quantitative assessment of the effect of drug therapy in improving ventricular function in cases of severe ventricular dysfunction secondary to

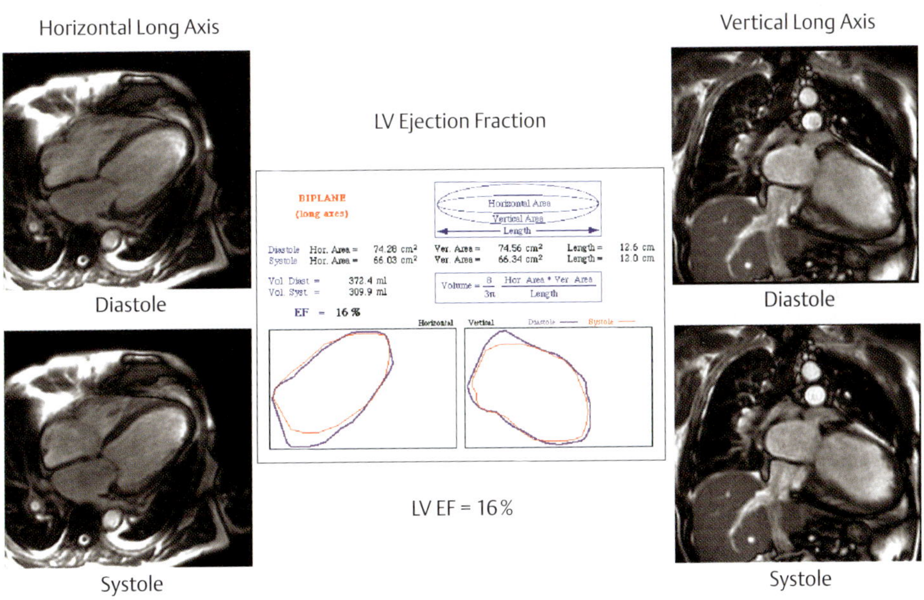

Fig. 7.**7** Global left ventricular hypokinesia and decrease in ejection fraction in a case of severe ischemic cardiomyopathy.

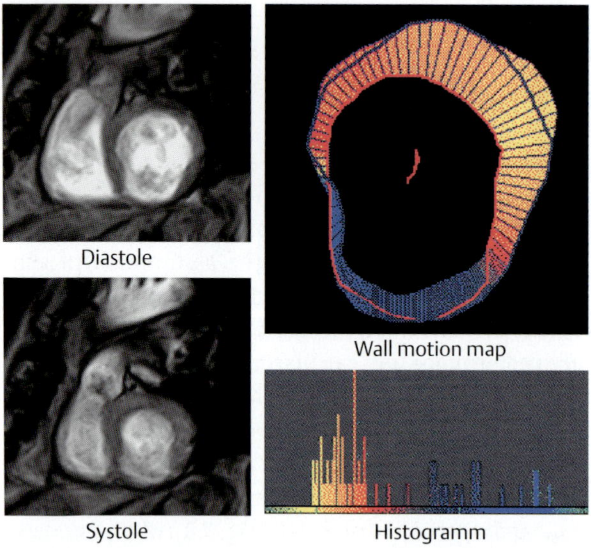

Fig. 7.**8** Quantitative evaluation of regional wall motion anomalies using sectorial analysis of the synchronicity of inward-outward ventricular motion depicting dyskinetic motion of the inferior wall in a different color scale. A histogram of distribution of different temporal parameters represents the disparity of regional asynchrony in wall motion.

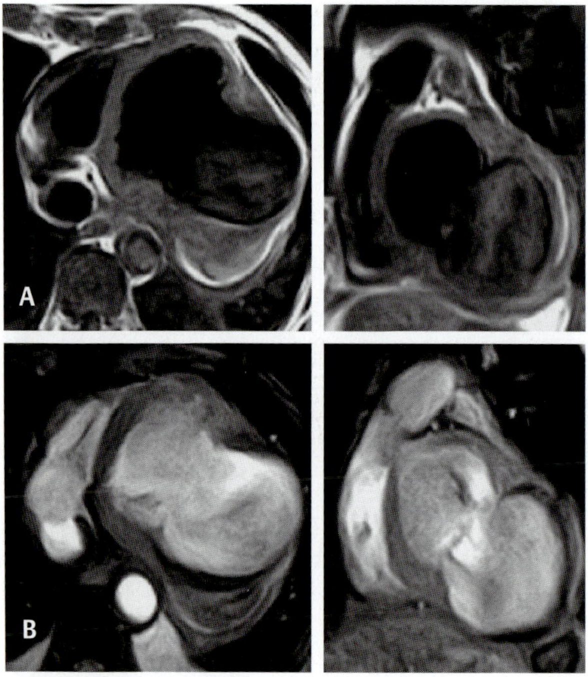

Fig. 7.**9** Development of a pseudoaneurysm following a myocardial rupture in a segment of myocardial infarction. (**A**) Spin-echo images show high signal intensity due to slow flow artifact. (**B**) Cine gradient-echo (GE) images show slow flow in the pseudoaneurysm.

severe ischemic cardiomyopathies or extended myocardial infarctions (Fig. 7.**9**). Although images acquired at rest provide adequate and relevant information in chronic ischemic disease, the identification of latent coronary disease with alterations occurring only during stress-induced ischemia require that images be acquired during pharmacologically-induced cardiovascular stress. Stress-induced regional or global myocardial wall motion anomalies are the most dependable indirect sign of insufficient coronary flow reserve and, therefore, of hemodynamically significant coronary disease.

7.2.2 Dobutamine Stress Test of Cardiac Function

Dobutamine stress testing is commonly used in combination with echocardiography and nuclear cardiography procedures for the evaluation of coronary artery disease by means of detection of wall motion abnormalities under pharmacological stress. Wall motion abnormalities can be induced in coronary beds fed by arteries with subcritical but hemodynamically significant stenosis. This situation occurs when the coronary reserve is insufficient to increase blood flow to match increased oxygen demand during pharmacological stress. Detection of induced wall motion abnormalities with high dose Dobutamine echocardiography (0–40 µg/kg per minute) has been shown to have a sensitivity of 83% and specificity of 85% for detection of ischemic heart disease. Unfortunately, transthoracic echocardiography is limited in image quality and 10 to 15% of Dobutamine studies are considered "technically poor" and studies are often unsuccessful due to the lack of an adequate acoustic window. MR imaging provides consistently superior image quality and has the added advantage of better myocardial-to-blood differentiation. Furthermore, the use of image tagging provides a more accurate quantitative motion evaluation that allows the detection of subtle wall motion abnormalities.

7.3 Assessment of Myocardial Perfusion and Viability

7.3.1 Quantitative Evaluation of Myocardial Perfusion

During the past decade, numerous clinical trials have demonstrated that contrast-enhanced myocardial perfusion MR imaging can provide a reliable investigative tool comparable to nuclear medicine studies in the evaluation of myocardial blood flow at rest and during stress (Fig. 7.**10**). In addition, MR perfusion images provide higher spatial and temporal resolution than conventional nuclear medicine imaging techniques, allowing for a higher sensitivity in depicting small regional perfusion anomalies and a better differentiation between subendocardial and transmural perfusion abnormalities. The measurements can be repeated regularly without any adverse effects for the patient. The MR perfusion imaging can also be combined with the evaluation of global and regional wall motion and wall thickening. Furthermore, the MR perfusion measurements can be safely acquired during baseline conditions at rest and during pharmacologically induced stress and hyperemia.

Recent studies reported that quantitative analysis of MR perfusion data could significantly improve the sensitivity and the specificity of the technique. In prior cardiac

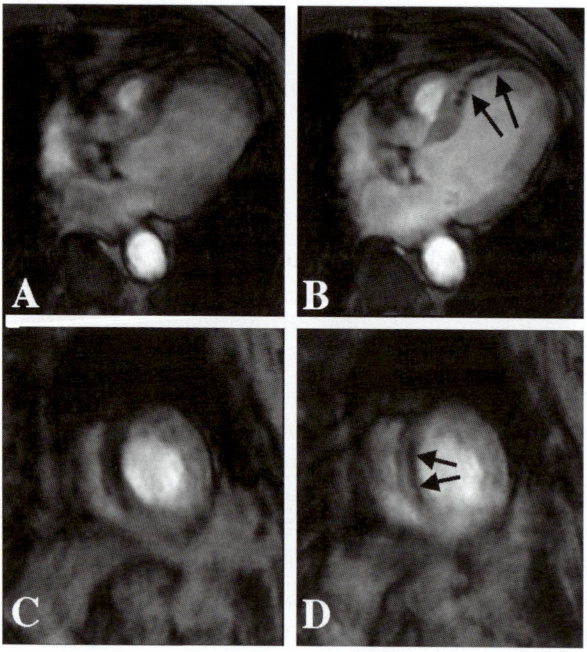

Fig. 7.10 Areas of low signal intensity in segments of hemorrhagic myocardial infarction pre- (**A** and **C**) and post-gadolinium injection (**B** and **D**).

nuclear studies the argument has been made that the addition of quantitative analysis in clinical routine may not improve significantly the diagnostic or prognostic value of a test but may help only to ameliorate the variability and bias of less experienced readers. This notion that quantitative analysis may not contribute significantly to the diagnostic value of cardiac nuclear testing may be partially due to the poor spatial resolution of the images and the high threshold for detecting relative perfusion changes in individual vascular beds. In MR perfusion imaging, however, recent data show a clear diagnostic benefit when quantitative analysis is applied. Even a semi-quantitative analysis of regional myocardial perfusion not only improves the sensitivity and specificity of the test but also allows better grading of coronary lesions. It is hypothesized that the extent and severity of myocardial injury and ischemia assessed using quantitative MR perfusion measurements will yield better outcome data and better risk stratification in patients with coronary artery disease.

7.3.2 Stress Testing of Myocardial Ischemia and Perfusion Reserve

Pharmacological stress testing using vasodilators such as dipyridamole or adenosine are used clinically as an alternative to exercise tests for the evaluation of stress-induced ischemia on myocardial perfusion tests in nuclear medicine. Recent clinical trials have demonstrated that similar stress testing can be applied to MR perfusion studies for the assessment of significance of coronary artery disease. A typical stress test using intravenous injection of adenosine at a dose of 140 µg/kg/min is applied to

MR perfusion imaging tests. Myocardial perfusion reserve can be evaluated regionally from rest and stress perfusion images. Different quantitative analysis techniques have been evaluated for a more quantitative measurement of regional alterations of myocardial perfusion. Compartmental models can be applied for the evaluation of myocardial contrast transit curve to determine regional blood flow. Simpler semiquantitative analysis techniques based on parameters such as peak signal enhancement, the maximum rate of enhancement during wash-in phase, or the time delay between bolus injection and peak signal enhancement in tissue have also been proposed. The validity and robustness of these parameters still need to be demonstrated in larger clinical trials [16].

MR perfusion imaging can be applied for assessing the severity and extent of perfusion alterations in coronary artery disease before and after interventions or for diagnostic purposes. It is hypothesized that a better and more accurate assessment of the extent and severity of myocardial jeopardy by quantitative measurements, will result in a better prediction of the outcome and the potential impact of a given therapeutic intervention. The ratio of measured myocardial blood flow at rest and during maximal hyperemia gives an estimate of the absolute and relative myocardial perfusion reserves. The perfusion reserve determined with MR perfusion imaging is a quantitative measure of the collateral-dependent myocardial flow. Preliminary clinical trials tend to demonstrate that MR perfusion imaging can help identify myocardial regions at risk and predict whether myocardial function may recover after myocardial infarction and revascularization. Another unique feature of MR perfusion imaging is its high spatial resolution and its ability to identify subendocardial perfusion defects as an early sign of ischemia, particularly in "hibernating" or "stunned" myocardium. The quantitative capabilities of MR perfusion imaging make this technique an ideal tool for following the effects of revascularization treatments irrespective of whether they are new minimal surgical interventions or new pharmaceutical strategies such as gene therapy.

7.3.3 Assessment of Myocardial Viability

Distinguishing between viable and non-viable myocardium is probably the most important clinical information supporting therapeutic decision making and patient management. Several MR imaging techniques have been applied in attempts to better predict myocardial viability, including MR spectroscopy, regional wall motion analysis and contrast-induced late myocardial enhancement [17]. Spectroscopic applications remain limited due to insufficient special and temporal resolution of these techniques. It is also well established that impaired myocardial contractility and regional wall motion abnormalities do not necessary represent irreversible tissue injury. Although regions of contractile dysfunction are often secondary to myocardial infarction and therefore irreversible, it is known that contractile dysfunction may also occur in viable myocardium and exhibit reversible improvement in function after reperfusion [18]. Following a transient ischemic event, for example, myocardial stunning may result in regional contractile alterations for prolonged periods of time. Similarly, chronic reductions in blood flow are thought to lead to myocardial hibernation, a state in which coronary blood supply is adequate to sustain viable myocytes but not to support contraction. The observation that the ejection fraction and regional alterations improve following revascularization in approximately one third of the patients with ischemic cardiomyopathy underscores that dysfunctional but viable myocardium is relatively common in clinical setting [19].

It has been well demonstrated that regions of myocardial injury exhibit higher signal intensity that does the normal myocardium on T2-weighted MR images without contrast agent enhancement and T1-weighted images following injection of contrast agent. Several recent studies performed in animal models and in clinical trials confirmed that areas of hyperenhancement represent irreversible myocardial damage. In a canine model, after varying length of coronary occlusion and reperfusion, the size and three-dimensional shape of hyperenhancement correlated closely with irreversible damage defined by ex vivo staining techniques [20]. In clinical trials in patients with ischemic ventricular dysfunction, segments showing transmural enhancement before revascularization showed less improvement in myocardial contractility after coronary revascularization than did areas without transmural or non-transmural enhancement [21]. Although the exact mechanism of gadolinium retention in areas of irreversible damage remains largely unknown, it is hypothesized that contrast uptake and wash-out kinetics as well as altered myocytes and sarcolemmal membrane integrity may play an important role [22,23].

7.4 Imaging of Coronary Arteries

7.4.1 Advances in Coronary Imaging Techniques

Direct visualization of coronary anatomy and coronary artherosclerotic stenosis is a determining parameter for definitive diagnosis and treatment of coronary artery disease. Not only is coronary angiography critical in identification of the location and severity of coronary stenosis, it is also necessary for the planning of therapeutic interventions such as revascularization or bypass surgery. Magnetic resonance coronary angiography has been demonstrated using a variety of imaging strategies. Most are designed and adapted to overcome one or more of the main inherent problems in coronary imaging:

- Motion of coronary arteries due to cardiac motion,
- Motion of coronary arteries due to respiratory motion,
- Signal to noise ratio,
- Contrast between coronary blood and surrounding tissues.

Although tremendous advances in MR coronary angiography were made during the past decade showing promising potential for non-invasive diagnosis of coronary ar-

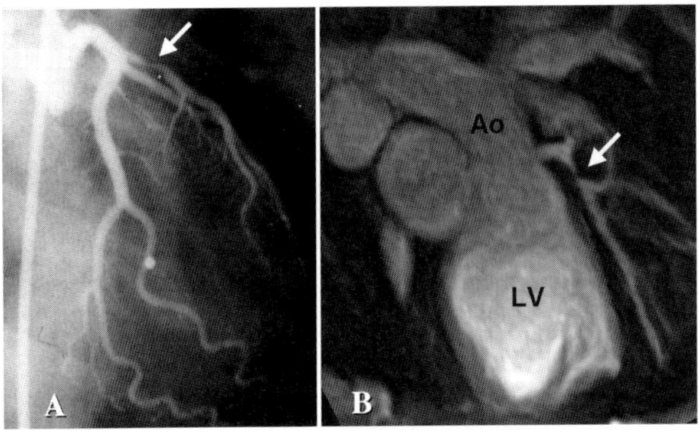

Fig. 7.**11** Example of coronary artery stenosis of the LAD depicted by (**A**) MR coronary angiography and (**B**) conventional X-ray contrast angiography.

tery disease, the clinical application of these techniques are still limited. The in-plane resolution of most current coronary MR imaging techniques is about 1 mm, sufficient for detection of stenosis in large coronary arteries but inadequate for accurate detection of disease in smaller branches of the coronary vasculature (Fig. 7.**11**). In vivo coronary angiography is particularly challenging, largely as a result of image artifacts and misregistration caused by cardiac and respiratory motion. Although cardiac motion artifacts can be effectively reduced by proper cardiac electrographic gating, compensation for respiratory motion represents a significantly greater challenge. The difficulties associated with respiratory motion artifacts are related to the fact that, unlike cardiac motion, respiratory motion of the diaphragm is highly irreproducible. Also a complete coronary angiogram requires sampling the entire heart, which is difficult to achieve within a single breath-hold. After numerous studies applying non-contrast 2D and 3D MR angiography techniques, the use of contrast-enhanced MRA for coronary imaging is emerging as a technique of choice, providing higher signal-to-noise ratio, higher contrast and higher spatial resolution. Contrast-enhanced MR angiography of the peripheral vasculature has gained increased clinical acceptance in the past few years showing significant improvements in image quality and diagnostic accuracy. Coronary angiograms can benefit from such improvements in imaging technique. With gadolinium injection the contrast is being generated by T1 differences and not in-flow dependence, hence larger volumes can be scanned without blood saturation. This means that 3D acquisition techniques with smaller isotropic voxels could be used, improving thereby the spatial resolution and the accuracy of detection of coronary stenoses. Using extracellular contrast agent a short T1 of the coronary arteries can be achieved only during the first pass of the contrast across the coronary vessels. However, since the contrast agent also diffuses into the interstitial space, it will also lower the T1 of the myocardium. Using this type of contrast agent limits the total acquisition time and therefore may limit the total number of slices that can be acquired. It is therefore suggested that intravascular contrast agents with a long blood half-life would improve the possibilities of MR imaging of coronary arteries.

7.4.2 Evaluation of Coronary Bypass Grafts

The MR imaging techniques developed for imaging coronary arteries have also been applied to imaging of coronary bypass grafts. MRI of proximal graft segments is usually easier than that of distal segments or native coronary arteries, because the former are less subject to cardiac motion and are not embedded in fat or in direct contact with the myocardium [24]. Most of the clinical studies available report on imaging of proximal vein grafts. Only a minority address MRI applicability in evaluating distal graft segments and arterial grafts, most likely because of the difficulty in obtaining adequate image quality, due to the artifacts associated with the abundant use of metallic hemostatic clips in internal mammary artery grafts. Also vein grafts are larger and therefore easier to image than arterial grafts [25].

So far, MR angiography of coronary bypass grafts has been limited to demonstrating the patency versus total occlusion only. Evidence in documenting non-occlusive graft disease has not been provided with the techniques used to date. Even a clear demonstration of graft patency or narrowing will often not suffice for clinical decision making. In most patients, there is also a need to know the status of the native coronary arteries. Clinical applications of MR angiography of bypass grafts are therefore limited to patients in whom there is no immediate need for knowing the status of the native coronary arteries. This category of patients includes patients with chest pain shortly after CABG surgery. Also, late after CABG surgery, information on whether the grafts are patent might be helpful in deciding to postpone coronary angiography in patients with ambiguous thoracic pain or mild anginal complaints. Non-invasive monitoring of flow parameters may also be useful to detect a gradual increase of graft stenosis and decide to proceed to X-ray angiography. Furthermore, MRI can be used as a screening procedure before angiography, indicating the number of grafts to be visualized and thereby shorten the angiographic procedure.

7.4.3 Measurement of Coronary Flow

Flow velocity and volume flow can be measured in coronary bypass grafts by applying velocity-encoded phase contrast cine MR sequences (see Chapter 1 for details on this technique). The quantitative evaluation of flow velocity allows the assessment of the functional characteristics of the graft in addition to a morphologic evaluation. Recent studies demonstrated that velocity profiles can be obtained in coronary grafts throughout the cardiac cycle in 85% of angiographically patent vein grafts using non-breath-hold MR velocity mapping [26]. Graft flow velocity was characterized by a biphasic pattern, with one peak in systole and a second peak in diastole. These findings match the observations obtained from invasive intracoronary Doppler guidewire measurements as well as transthoracic Doppler echocardiography. More recently, breath-hold segmented k-space sequences have been applied to measure flow velocity and volume flow at rest and after pharmacological stress. Using non-breath-hold and breath-hold techniques, functional results were also obtained in IMA grafts, despite the imaging artifacts due to metallic clips.

7.5 References

1. Grover-McKay M, Bradley WG, Jr. Technological advances make cardiovascular MRI a clinical reality. Diagnostic Imaging 2001; 61–67.
2. Ratib O, Didier D, Chatelain P, Righetti A, Lerch R, Townsend D. Standard views in cardiac multimodality tomographic imaging. Am J Card Imaging 1995; 9: 67–76.
3. Didier D, Ratib O, Friedli B, et al. Cine gradient-echo MR imaging in the evaluation of cardiovascular diseases. RadioGraphics 1993; 13: 561–573.
4. Reichek N. MRI Myocardial tagging. J Magn Reson Imaging 1999; 10: 609–616.
5. Wilke N, Jerosch-Herold M, Zenovich A, Stillman A. Magnetic resonance first-pass myocardial perfusion imaging: Clinical validation and future applications. J Magn Reson Imaging 1999; 10: 676–685.
6. Sechtem U, Baer F, Voth E, Theissen P, Schneider C. Stress functional MRI: Detection of ischemic heart disease and myocardial viability. J Magn Reson Imaging 1999; 10: 667–675.
7. Lim T-H, Choi SI. MRI of myocardial infarction. J Magn Reson Imaging 1999; 10: 686–693.
8. Ramani K, Judd RM, Holly TA, et al. Contrast magnetic resonance imaging in the assessment of myocardial viability in patients with stable coronary artery disease and left ventricular dysfunction. Circulation 1998; 98: 2687–2694.
9. Simonetti OP, Kim RJ, Fieno DS, et al. An improved MRI technique for visualization of myocardial infarction. Radiology 2001; 218: 215–223.
10. Wendland M, Saeed M, Lund G, Higgins C. Contrast-enhanced MRI for quantification of myocardial viability. J Magn Reson Imaging 1999; 10: 694–702.
11. Yeh B. Magnetic resonance imaging of the coronary arteries. Applied Radiology Supplement 2000; April: 68–75.
12. Duerinckx AJ, Atkinson DP, Mintorovitch J, Simonetti OP, Vrman MK. Two dimensional coronary MRA: limitations and artifacts. Eur Radiology 1996; 6: 312–325.
13. Botnar R, Stuber M, Danias P, Kissinger, Kraig, Manning W. A fast 3D approach for coronary MRA. J Magn Reson Imaging 1999; 10: 821–825.
14. Duerinckx AJ, Atkinson DP, Hurwitz R. Assessement of coronary artery patency after stent placement using magnetic resonance angiography. J. Magn Reson Imaging 1998; 8: 896–902.
15. Li D, Kaushikkar S, Haacke EM, et al. Coronary arteries: three-dimensional MR imaging with retrospective respiratory gating. Radiology 1996; 201: 857–863.
16. Vallee J-P, MacFall J, Lazeyras F, et al. Pitfalls in myocardial perfusion assessment with dynamic MR imaging after administration of a contrast material bolus in dogs. Academic Radiology 1999: 512–520.

17. Fieno DS, Kim RJ, Chen EL, Lomasney JW, Klocke FJ, Judd RM. Contrast-enhanced magnetic resonance imaging of myocardium at risk: Distinction between reversible and irreversible injury throughout infarct healing. J Am Coll Cardiol 2000; 36: 1985–1991.
18. Kroft L, Doornbos J, van der Geest R, Benderbous S, de Roos A. Infarcted myocardium in pigs: MR imaging enhanced with slow-interstitial-diffusion gadolinium compound P760. Radiology 1999; 212: 467–473.
19. Kim R, Wu E, Rafael A, et al. The use of contrast-enhanced magnetic resonance imaging to identify reversible myocardial dysfunction. New Engl J Med 2000; 343: 1445–1453.
20. Klein C, Nekolla S, Bengel F, et al. Assessment of myocardial viability with contrast-enhanced magnetic resonance imaging; comparison with positron emission tomography. Circulation 2002; 105: 162–167.
21. Kim RJ, Fieno DS, Parrish TB, et al. Relationship of MRI delayed contrast enhancement to irreversible injury, infarct age, and contractile function. Circulation 1999; 100: 1992–2002.
22. Hillenbrand HB, Kim RJ, Parker MA, Fieno DS, Judd RM. Early assessment of myocardial salvage by contrast-enhanced magnetic resonance imaging. Circulation 2000; 102: 1678–1683.
23. Saeed M, Bremerich J, Wendland M, Wyttenbach R, Weinmann H-J, Higgins C. Reperfused myocardial infarction as seen with use of necrosis-specific versus standard extracellular MR contrast media in rats. Radiology 1999; 213: 247–257.
24. van Rossum AC, Bedaux W, Hofman M. Morphologic and functional evaluation of coronary artery bypass conduits. 1999; 10: 734–740.
25. Galjee MA, van Rossum AC, Doesburg T, van Eenige MJ, Visser CA. Value of magnetic resonance imaging in assessing patency and function of coronary bypass grafts: an angiographically controlled study. Circulation 1996: 93: 660–666.
26. Kalden P, Kreitner KF, Wittlinger T, et. al. Assessment of coronary bypass grafts: value of different breath-hold MR imaging techniques. AJR 1999: 172: 1359–1264.

8 Index

A

B

C

D

N

P

R

S

9 Dynamic Cardiac MRI – Companion CD

9.1 System Requirements

9.1.1 Macintosh

- System 8.0 or later
- QuickTime extension (installed in standard Mac OS)
- 4 MB of free disk space
- CD ROM drive
- Minimum display resolution of 640 × 480 with 256 colors

9.1.2 Windows PC

- Microsoft Windows 98 or later
- QuickTime Player (provided on this CD)
- 4 MB of free disk space
- CD ROM drive
- Minimum display resolution of 640 × 480 with 256 colors

9.2 Installation

9.2.1 Macintosh

- Insert the disk in your CD ROM drive
- Wait for a few seconds, the program should start automatically
- If the program does not start automatically open the CD and double click on the file called **Start_Tour**
- Select the chapter that you want to review (see illustration below)

9.2.2 Windows PC

- Insert the disk in your CD ROM drive
- Wait for a few seconds, the program should start automatically
- If the program does not start automatically open the CD and double click on the file called **Start_Teaching_Tour.exe**
- Select the chapter that you want to review (see illustration below)

- **If the dynamic cine-sequences don't show up, you must install QuickTime viewer on your computer**. Go to the directory called QuickTime Installer and double click on QuickTime Installer

9.3 User Manual

After starting the program shows a list of different chapters to choose from:

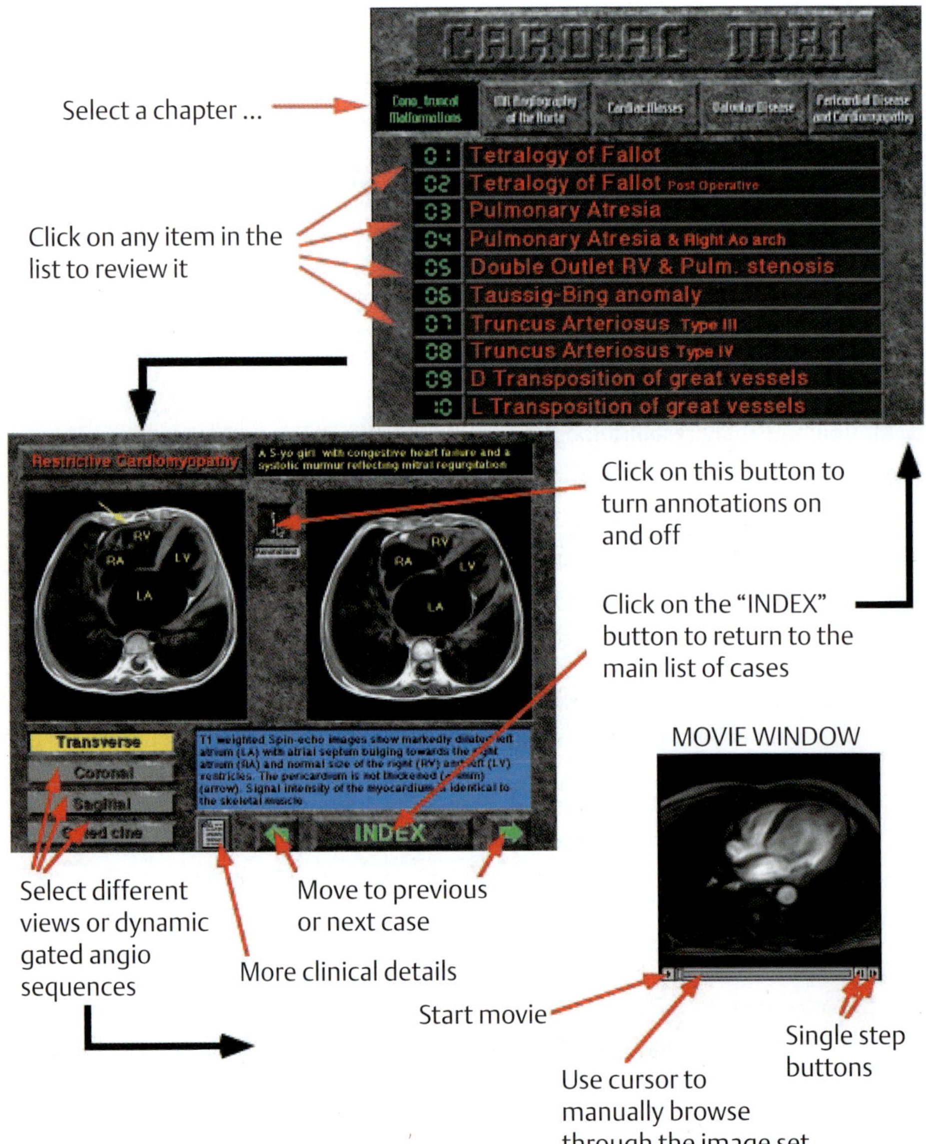